Luke Curtis, MD, MS, CIH
Medical Writer / Researcher
8469 Beech Avenue, Apart #2
Cincinnati, OH 45236

D0969431

Elder Nutrition

2-8-2011

DEAR HEIDI
   THANK FOR YOUR
SUPPORT OVER THE
YEARS. THIS BOOK HAS
GOOD SUGGESTIONS FOR
NON-ELDERLY LIKE
YOURSELF.

Love
   —Luke Curtis—
      847-769-4768

Elder Nutrition

HOW ADULTS IN THEIR SEVENTIES, EIGHTIES,
AND NINTIES CAN OBTAIN AND MAINTAIN GOOD HEALTH
AND STAY ACTIVE BY PROPER NUTRITION, EXERCISE,
SOCIAL SUPPORT, AND A POSITIVE MENTAL ATTITUDE

*A Practical and Optimistic Guide Based on Dr. Curtis's
Experience in Treating Hundreds of Elder Patients with
Nutritional Problems and Based on Hundreds of Recent
Published Studies on Nutritional Research*

Luke Curtis, MD

To order additional copies of this book, contact:
Xlibris Corporation
1-888-795-4274
www.Xlibris.com
Orders@Xlibris.com
75843

CONTENTS

DEDICATION

This book is devoted to my father, Herbert John Curtis (1918-2007). He inspired me for a love of both in reading and writing. Good nutrition allowed him to live to age 88 years in excellent health. He was killed at age 89 years after acquiring sixteen hospital-acquired infections following minor surgery.

ABOUT THE AUTHOR

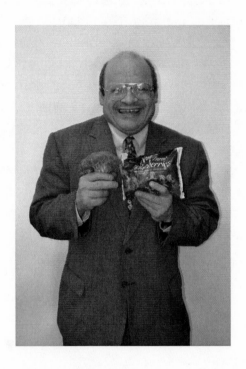

L uke Curtis, MD, MS, CIH is a physician and medical writer living in Chicago, Illinois. He has an MD from St. Christopher's Medical School in Lutom, Great Britain, and an MS in public health, magna cum laude, from the University of Illinois at Chicago. Luke also has a BS in biology and chemistry from Valparaiso University. Luke has completed eleven university level courses in nutrition and biochemistry. He has counseled and treated over one thousand patients on nutritional issues. Luke has written and published over sixty papers and articles in peer-reviewed medical journals on a wide range of topics including nutrition, allergy, infection control, occupational/ environmental medicine and indoor/outdoor air quality. He has also published over 150 articles on nutritional, environmental, and medical topics in the popular press. Dr. Curtis has also written regular medical articles and blogs for the past two years for Mediatrition (Rockwall, Texas) and for the past twenty years in the *Human Ecologist* (Atlanta, Georgia).

Luke Curtis has also done extensive paid and volunteer clinical work with residents of elder care facilities. Luke especially enjoys talking to older patients and learning more about life in the 1920s, 1930s, and 1940s. During his medical school days, Luke received an "Outstanding" grade for his work on a twelve-week geriatric internal medicine rotation.

Luke also has twenty years experience in public health. In 1995, Dr. Curtis was awarded a Centers for Disease Control (CDC) Commendation for Exceptional Performance for his work in leading a Chicago investigation of lung hemorrhage in infants.

ABOUT THE ILLUSTRATOR

J enn Wilson is a professor at Columbia College in Chicago and the School of the Art Institute in Chicago. She teaches painting, drawing, and art history courses. She received her MFA from The School of the Art Institute in Chicago and her BFA at Washington University in Saint Louis She is also an artist and shows her work in several galleries in Chicago. Jenn Wilson received a Cushing Grant in 2004 and a School of the Art Institute of Chicago Travel Grant to Italy in 2002. Jenn was also Artist in Residence at the Badlands National Park in 2006, and was a Union League Arts Council Finalist in 2008.

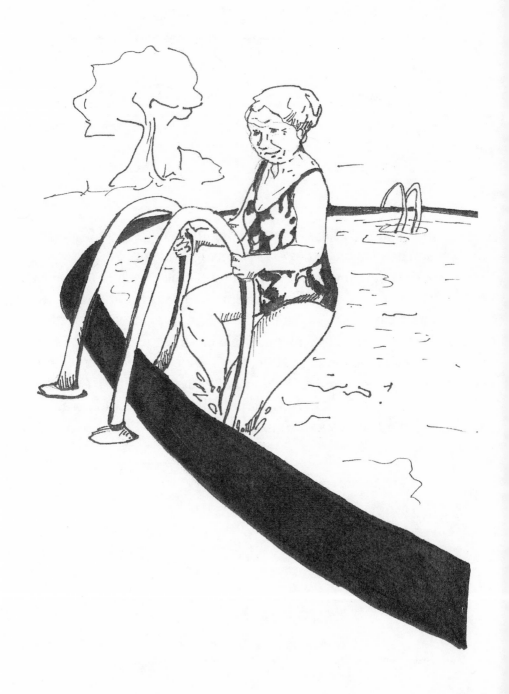

CHAPTER 1

INTRODUCTION: SENIORS ARE A GROWING AND VITAL PART OF THE POPULATION WHOSE QUALITY OF LIFE IS OFTEN IMPAIRED BY NUTRITIONAL PROBLEMS

The Senior Population Is Growing Very Rapidly

Persons older than 65 or 70 years represent the largest growing segment of the population of the USA, Canada, and most of the developing nations. In the USA, the number of people older than 65 years is expected to more than double from 35 million in 2010 to 71 million in 2030 (US Census 2008). In just the 20 years between 2010 and 2030, the number of US citizens over age 80 years is expected to more than double from 9 million to 19.5 million (US Census 2008).

The numbers of people older than 90 years is also expected to increase rapidly. The number of US residents older than 90 years was 1.5 million in 2000 and is expected to rise to about 2.3 million by 2010 (US Census 2001). Financial planners are now urging couples in their sixties to plan for a long retirement. Among a married couple aged 65 years, there is a 45% chance that one or both will live till 90 or older (Society of Actuaries 2000).

Centenarians, or people over 100 years old, are also increasing rapidly. In 2007, Hallmark Cards printed 86,000 birthday cards for people of over 100 years (Bailik 2008). The 2000 US Census reported 82,000 US citizens over the age of 100 years. The number of US citizens over 100 years old is expected to grow to 126,000 by 2010 and to 1.1 million by 2050 (Bailik 2008). In 2007, the author's small church of only about 250 members had four members older than 100 years old. A British study estimated that if current trends continue, about 21% (more than one in five) Britons born in 2007 can expect to reach the 100-year mark (BBC 2007).

Seniors Are a Vital and Important Part of Society

Many seniors are still quite active in terms of work, community and religious service, exercise, gardening work, travel, and family and social activity. Some say that 70 years old is now considered the new 60 or even 50 years of age. Six million seniors over age 65 years (or about 20% of their population) are still employed in the US labor force, with about half of them employed full-time (US Bureau of Labor Statistics 2008). Over 1 million US citizens over age 75 years are still working (about 7% of their population) (US Bureau of Labor Statistics 2008). Thankfully, mandatory age retirement laws are being repealed in many states. The number of seniors in the workforce is expected to grow in the coming years as both longevity and economic problems increase. Many people are beginning second or third careers in a new line of work after age 65. Millions more seniors who are not employed in payroll jobs are either employed in volunteer positions or are self-employed.

Seniors are especially active in vital occupations such as farming and ranching. In 2008, 31% of all US farms were actively operated by farmers older than 65 years (USDA 2008). This author has learned a lot about raising agricultural crops and animals by talking to hundreds of seniors who are still involved in farming.

Elders make excellent teachers of just about any topic. The author recounts that many of his best teachers and professors were past 65 when he took their classes. During his first semester of undergraduate studies at Valparaiso University, four out of five of his professors were over 68 years of age. Many retired professors still continue doing valuable research, teaching, and mentoring past 70 years of age.

Older adults are often greatly involved in family life. About 23% of all US children under age of 5 are cared for during at least part of the week by grandparents (AARP 2009). Older adults are also often involved in caregiving of an ailing spouse, sibling, adult child, or even a very elderly parent/aunt/uncle. Many people's most cherished memories come from time spent with grandparents, great-aunts/uncles, and other older relatives.

Seniors are often quite active and play an indispensable role in many worthwhile volunteer activities such as religious activities, school tutoring, sports coaching, scouting, and fraternal organizations. For example, a 2002 ABC poll reported that 60% of US Christians over age 65 years attend church each Sunday, as compared to only 28% of those in the 18 to 30 year old age group (ABC 2002). Persons in the over 65 year old age groups on average also donate more time and money to church than any other age group (ABC 2002).

Elders represent the age group most likely to vote in local, state, and national elections. For example, in the 2008 US presidential election, 68% of adults over 65 years voted as compared to only 56% of all adults below the age of 65 years (US Census 2009). Seniors are often very politically active and, on average, contribute more time and money on political causes than any other age group.

Seniors are often involved in all sorts of interesting hobbies from bridge to gardening to stamp collecting to coaching. In college, the author won a cross-country letter for Valparaiso (Indiana) University in 1977. At several Indiana cross-country meets, our team met the De Pauw cross-country coach who was 88 years old and was still jogging 3 to 5 miles daily. Elders are frequently involved in gardening work and often do paid or volunteer landscaping work. The author developed his lifelong love of gardening mostly from his grandparents and older neighbors.

Many seniors successfully hold political office. Legislators over age 65 years comprise 24% of the 50 US state legislatures (NCSL 2009). In the US Congress, 14% of the legislators are over 70 years, and 34% are in the 60 to 69 year old age group (Congress.org 2009). Elders make up a large percentage of mayors and councilpersons in cities and towns. Senator Robert Byrd Jr. (1917-) of West Virginia is the US Senate president pro tem at age 92. Claude Pepper (1900-1989), who was both senator and congressman from Florida, was serving Congress as a very active advocate for seniors until he died at age 89. Many famous national leaders have led their nation successfully when past 75 years of age. Ronald Reagan (1911-2004) was president of the United States until age 77 years, and Winston Churchill (1874-1965) was prime minister of Britain at age 80. Konrad Adenauer (1876-1967) was chancellor for fourteen years when he led West Germany's amazing World War II-postwar economic recovery (*Wirtschaftswunder* or "Economic Miracle") at age 73 to 87 years. President Nelson Mandela (1918-) led South Africa through its post-apartheid period until age 80. Golda Meir (1898-1978) was prime minister of Israel at age 76.

Besides politics, many people older than 75 years have done many great things in many fields including medicine, science, arts, and social activism. Alice Hamilton, MD (1869-1970), was the mother of modern occupational medicine and the first female professor at Harvard. Alice was still quite active well into her eighties. Mary Harris "Mother" Jones (1830-1930) was a

LUKE CURTIS, MD

prominent labor and community organizer who was active well into her nineties. Anna "Grandma" Moses (1860-1961) took up painting in her seventies and worked almost up to her death at age 101 producing 3,600 wonderful paintings. The great German author Johann Wolfgang von Goethe (1749-1832) completed his masterwork *Faust* when aged 80 years. Connie Mack (1862-1956) was still actively managing the Philadelphia Athletics major league baseball team until age 87. Pablo Picasso (1881-1973) produced hundreds of paintings past the age of 85. Arthur Fieldler (1894-1979) conducted the Boston Pops Orchestra actively for 50 years until his death at age 84. Norman Borlaug (1914-2009), winner of the 1970 Nobel Peace Prize for developing higher-yielding strains of wheat and rice, continued his agricultural research and activism well into his eighties. Mother Teresa of Calcutta (1910-1997), who won the Nobel Peace Prize in 1979 for her work with the poor of India, was active in her humanitarian activities until almost her death at age 87.

Our present world would be a much poorer place in many ways without the many contributions of many people in their senior years. Improved nutrition will enable many elder people to remain active for more years and contribute a lot of wonderful things to society.

While many older adults could benefit from more exercise, many older adults are still active physically in a wide range of sports. A US survey found that the 69% of adults aged 65 to 74 years and 60% of adults over age 75 years met the minimum recommended exercise levels of at least thirty minutes of moderate activity (such as walking at 3 miles per hour) for at least five times per week (AQHRQ 2000). The ten most popular sports for seniors include walking, stretching, use of treadmills and stationary bikes, golf, bowling, swimming, fishing, weight lifting, gardening, and camping (Superstudy 1999). Some seniors are more active than most younger adults and compete in long-distance walking, jogging, bicycling, and swimming; dance competitively; play "mean" games of tennis or golf; or work at physically demanding jobs like farming. In 2008, the author rode his bike 104 miles in a single day in a group of cyclists that included a 90-year-old retired high school teacher. The 90-year-old teacher was still in fairly good health except for being hard of hearing and having a slight tremor. Some of the research on the benefits of exercise on senior health will be mentioned in following chapters.

Over 22 million people over age 65 years had US driver's licenses in 2003 (Messenger 2003). Persons are frequently driving well into their eighties and nineties. Driving is often seen as an important factor in personal independence. Many new communities make the ability to drive almost essential for getting around as no public transportation is provided, and work, family and friends homes, and shopping, religious, medical and recreational activities are widely dispersed. Moreover, the physical layout of many new communities discourages walking and bicycling in several ways, including providing no sidewalks or streetlights and not providing a grid street pattern but instead funneling all traffic into high-speed, high-traffic arterial roads.

Statistically speaking, the safest drivers are those in the 50 to 75 year old age group. After age 75 years, seniors start to have increased rates of both traffic accidents and traffic related deaths (Messenger 2003). Many states such as Illinois require that senior motorists take vision and driving tests more frequently than younger drivers. The author knows of one case in which an 83-year-old neighbor fell asleep while driving and crashed into a jewelry store. Thankfully, no one was seriously hurt.

Older adults often enjoy frequent vacation travel if their health and finances permit. Elders have the highest travel rates of any age group. A US Travel Industry Association survey reported that those over 55 years old took 179 million trips for business and pleasure in 1999. This represents over 31% of the trips taken by people of all ages (US TIA 1999). Many packaged tours and cruises are geared primarily to older adults. "Grandtravel" or

LUKE CURTIS, MD

grandparents traveling with grandchildren on vacation trips is becoming increasingly common. About 21% of all vacation trips taken with children involve one or more grandparents (American Demographics 2001).

Many seniors are still involved in close romantic relationships. In 1996, over 2.6 million US couples have been married fifty years or more to celebrate their golden wedding anniversary (US Census 1996). In 2009, Herbert (age 104) and Zelmyra (age 101) Fisher of New Bern, North Carolina, have been happily married for eighty-five years. They are both still in fairly good health, living in their own home, and attending church every Sunday. They were recognized by the Guinness Book of World Records as having the world record for the longest marriage (Hendricks 2009). Other seniors are still dating and remarrying. In 2003, about 13% of the people who wed were over 45 years old, and 4% were over 65 years old (Jayson 2008). Many new dating services are opening, which cater largely or exclusively to older folks. For example the dating site Match.com has 2.5 million members over the age of 55 (webpersonals.online 2009).

Many seniors are still sexually active past 70. A survey of 3,005 older US reports found that 53% of those 65 to 74 years and 26% of those over age 75 years were still sexually active (Lindau 2007). A study of 70-year-olds in Sweden reported that 68% of men and 56% of women with spouses/partners reported regular sexual intercourse (Beckman 2008). The author remembers from his medical school days talking to a man of 91 years and a woman of 88 years. The man had been a paratrooper in France on D-day, while the woman had taught school for over forty years. This couple had been dating each other for two years after they each lost their beloved spouses after more than sixty years of happy marriage. The 88-year-old woman insisted her boyfriend take Viagra (sildenafil) so they could have a better sex life. Subsequent visits by this couple indicated that the Viagra was effective. Another couple the author met during medical school was both 91 years old, married for seventy-one years and reported having "wonderful" sex two to three times per week. The husband told me that extended and thorough foreplay was the key to excellent sex in the later years. On the negative side, many elders would like to remain sexually intimate but do not have a spouse or partner.

Many Seniors Are Plagued by Nutrition Related Health Problems Which Impair Their Quality of Life

Although many seniors have very active and fulfilling lives, many are plagued with many chronic health problems that limit their ability to function. Nutrition plays a key role in preventing or treating many serious acute and chronic health conditions including heart disease, stroke, asthma and allergies, kidney disease, vision problems, digestive problems, diabetes, joint problems, chronic fatigue, and many forms of cancer. Nutrition also plays an important role in preventing mental depression, preventing or slowing down loss of mental functions (dementia), and preventing or slowing the loss of bone and muscle with age. Proper nutrition can also reduce the risk of many infections, including many life-threatening hospital-acquired infections. Proper nutrition can often mean the difference between death and a good recovery to those undergoing major surgery, cancer, heart attack, or stroke or for patients unfortunate enough to wind up in intensive care units. The effects of nutrition on preventing and treating common diseases will be described in detail in the following chapters.

In spite of the obvious health benefits of good nutrition, more than half of all seniors have significant nutritional deficiencies. The second chapter of this book will describe how common elder malnutrition is and what are the reasons for these nutritional problems.

I am writing this book to promote better nutrition and nutritional awareness among older folks and their families and caregivers. While there are many popular books about nutrition, very few have focused on the nutritional needs of older adults. Experience and research show that many of their chronic health problems are due less to the aging process than to the malnutrition that occurs in a majority of seniors. The purpose of this book is to help seniors avoid or mitigate chronic health problems and lead a longer and more active and fulfilling life through improved nutrition and other factors such as sleep, exercise, social activities, and positive mental attitude. Providing better nutrition for US seniors will also save many billions of dollars in health care and disability costs.

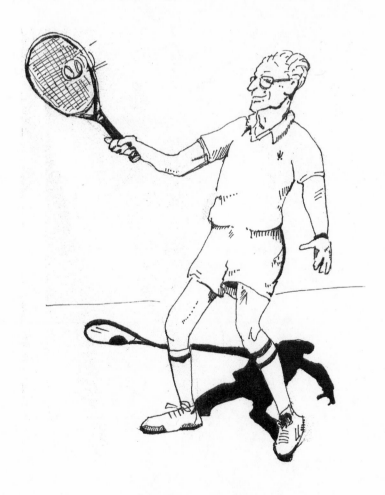

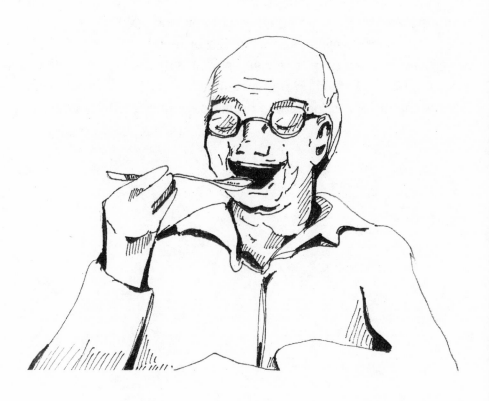

CHAPTER 2

MOST OLDER ADULTS ARE MALNOURISHED, WHY?

Extent of Malnutrition in Seniors

Many older adults are not getting the nutrition they need to maintain optimum health. This is even true of many adults who were healthy and well-nourished in middle age. This second chapter will report the extent of malnutrition among seniors and examine why poor nutrition is so common in older adults.

Many Elders Deficient in Protein, Calories and Water

Just how common is malnutrition among older adults? The answer largely depends upon how malnutrition is defined. In the most obvious forms of malnutrition, elders are often deficient in protein, calories, or water. People with deficiencies in protein and calories are often low in blood proteins such as albumin, transferritin, or prealbumin. Lack of protein and calories cause rapid loss of bone and muscle mass and greatly increases risk of infection and death (Price 2008). The need for calories and proteins varies somewhat due to body size and activity levels. It is recommended that a moderately active 70-year-old weighing about 74 kilograms (162 pounds) consume about 2,000 kCalories of energy and at least 60 grams a day of protein (Whitney 2008).

Protein/calorie malnutrition is very common in US seniors living at home and in elder care and hospital facilities. One survey reported that at least 16% of adults over 65 years living at home had severe protein and calorie malnutrition (Merck 2006). One review of five large studies of older hospitalized patients reported that 42% to 91% have severe deficiencies of protein and calories (Kubrak and Jensen 2007).

Another common form of malnutrition in seniors is dehydration. Most authorities recommend that seniors consume at least six to ten eight-ounce glasses of liquid (which includes water, soup, milk, juice, smoothies, coffee, tea, etc.) per day, depending upon body size, activity, and temperature. Many seniors do not get enough water and other liquids in their diet and often become dehydrated. The risk of dehydration is especially high during hot weather (sweating) or when people lost fluids from diarrhea, vomiting, or blood loss (Morley 2009). Estimates on the extent of dehydration in people over 70 years old varies widely and ranges from a 0.5% rate of severe dehydration to a 60% rate of mild dehydration (Stookey 2005). Seniors often have a reduced thirst drive in the brain and must be encouraged to drink more fluids in the day (Schols 2009). Neglect in nursing homes also frequently causes serious dehydration (Sullivan 2005). Dehydration can increase risk of many serious health problems including heart and kidney problems, difficulty in breathing, infections and increase risk of catastrophic low blood pressure or shock.

Most Elders Lacking in Many Vitamins, Minerals and Omega-3 Fats

In addition to inadequate nutrition in terms of protein, calories, and fluids, most US seniors simply do not consume enough of many vitamins, minerals, fatty acids, proteins, and many other vital nutrients in their regular diets. For example, various studies have reported that the average 60-plus person in the USA consumes only 20% of the United States Food and Drug Administration Recommended Daily Allowances (USRDA) for vitamin D, 55% of the USRDA for vitamin E, 60% of the USRDA for calcium, and 75% of the USRDA for vitamin K (Park 2008). Average magnesium consumption among women over 65 years is only 68% of the USRDA (Rude 2009). Other studies involving elderly adults in developed nations have reported that average intake of zinc is only about 60% of USRDA and average intake of potassium is only about 50% of USRDA (Prasad 1993; Gorelik 2003). A survey of 4,805 adults in all fifty US states and DC reported that 46% do not consume the recommended USRDA daily minimum of 60 milligrams of vitamin C (Taylor 2000). In developed nations such as the United States, Europe, and Australia, the average consumption of omega-3 fatty acids is less than one-third of the recommended level of 3.2 grams per day (Meyer 2003).

Many elders show deficiencies of nutrients when given tests of blood or urine. Deficiencies of vitamins D, B_{12}, folate, and calcium are especially common in elders. One huge study of 3,170 US adults over age 60 years reported that vitamin D deficiency was found in 76% of whites, 96% of blacks, and 92% of Mexican Americans! (Ginde 2009). Among a group of 548 nonhospitalized elderly US adults (average age of 77 range of 67 to 96 years), 40.5% had blood deficiencies of vitamin B_{12} (cobalamin), and 23.5% have blood deficiencies of folate (Lindenbaum 1994). Inadequate calcium intake from food and huge losses from calcium in bones are found in a majority of elders. Calcium deficiencies are often present in seniors even if blood calcium levels appear "normal" (Park2008). Other studies have reported that a large percentage of seniors have low blood and tissue levels of important minerals such as magnesium, zinc, chromium, and selenium (Vaquero 2002).

Inadequate Consumption of Fruits and Vegetables

A majority of seniors and people of all ages do not consume enough fruits and vegetables. Daily consumption of five to ten one-half-cup servings of a wide range of fruits and vegetables is critical for maintaining good health. Vegetables and fruits are rich in water, fiber, and minerals and vitamins. Fruits and vegetables also contain a wide variety of plant-synthesized chemicals called "phytochemicals", which fight heart disease, strokes, cancer, infection, allergy, and many other health problems. Many later chapters of this book will discuss the health benefits of fruits and vegetables in detail.

The US Department of Health and Human Services recommends all adults eat at least two fruit servings and three vegetables servings each day (US Dept. of Health and Human Services 2000). The American Cancer Society recommends that all adults consume at least five servings of fruits and vegetables daily and preferably more (Byers 2002). However, most people of all ages do not get the recommended 5 ½-cup servings of fruits and vegetables per day. A nationwide survey of 72,253 US adults over age 65 reported that only 45% eat two or more servings a day of fruit and a mere 33% consume the recommended three or more servings a day of vegetables (MMWR 2007). Not getting the recommended quantities of fruits and vegetables can increase risk for heart disease, high blood pressure, many cancers, loss of mental function (dementia), and eye problems. The relationship between fruit and vegetable consumption in preventing, or at least slowing progression of many diseases, will be discussed in many of the following chapters.

It is important to realize that the nutritional needs of seniors may vary considerably from person to person depending upon a number of factors including (1) how well they absorb food, (2) what health problems they have, and (3) genetic factors. For optimum health, many seniors may have to consume more than the US recommended daily allowance for protein and certain vitamins and minerals. Later chapters will give specific recommendations as to the types of food to consume and the types and quantities of food supplements to take.

Many researchers feel that the US Recommended Daily Allowances for many nutrients such as vitamins C and D are too low and need to be increased to allow for optimum nutrition (Deruelle 2008; Linnebur 2007).

Why Malnutrition Is So Common among US Seniors

Why is malnutrition so common among elders? There are many reasons, which include problems with chewing, swallowing, and digesting food; lower daily food consumption; less food variety; poorer absorption of food; chronic illnesses; poverty; drug use; heavy alcohol consumption; mental depression; and death or chronic illness of spouse or other family members. Oftentimes, a combination of these factors will turn an adult who was well nourished in middle age to an elderly adult with many nutritional deficiencies.

Swallowing and Tooth/Denture Problems Reduce Nutrient Intake

Problems with swallowing and/or problems with teeth/dentures can reduce food intake in elders. Difficulties in swallowing, or dysphasia, affect about 15% of seniors living at home and about 40% of those living in elder care facilities (Humbert 2008). About 40% of the US population over age 75 years has a complete set of dentures (Douglass 2000).

Problems with sense of smell and taste have become much more common after age 70 years and can greatly reduce appetite and food intake in elders (Murphy 2008).

Digestive Problems Make Eating Uncomfortable

Digestive problems and digestive discomfort can also greatly reduce nutritional intake.

Digestive problems such as stomach acid reflux (heartburn), stomach or intestinal ulcers, bowel incontinence (inability to control bowel movements), constipation, diarrhea, irritable bowel syndrome, or chronic intestinal infections like *Closteridium difficile* are much more common in elders than middle-aged folk (Crane 2007). In US adults over age 65 years, the prevalence of heartburn is about 10-20%, discomfort from stomach or intestinal ulcers about 9%, and presence irritable bowel syndromes (abdominal pain, chronic diarrhea, chronic constipation, or any combination of this three) is about 6-18% (Crane 2007). The chronic diarrhea seen in irritable bowel syndrome or chronic intestinal infections like *Closteridium difficile* show significant amounts of water and other nutrients being consumed and cause dehydration (loss of water) and deficiencies in many nutrients such as protein, fat, calories, and many vitamins and minerals (Morley 2009). All of these digestive problems can reduce food intake and make eating and/or bowel movements very uncomfortable. For more information about treating digestive problems in the elderly, please see chapter 13.

Poverty and Lack of Readily Available Healthy Food Limit Nutrition

Poverty is a major factor in promoting malnutrition. In 2007, 10% of the US adults over aged 65 years lived below the poverty level (US Administration on Aging 2008). About 60% of poor elders are not taking advantage of federal and state food assistance programs like the Supplemental Nutrition Assistance Program (SNAP) they are entitled to. The author encourages all low-income readers to apply for government food assistance programs. Several studies have reported that participation in government food programs is associated with significantly less hunger and better overall nutrition (Nelson 1998).

Many studies have reported that poverty in older adults is associated with lower consumption of many nutrients and healthy foods such as fruits, vegetables, meats, fish, and low-fat dairy products (Sharkey 2008; Nelson 1998). Poverty can force many seniors to live on cheap diets rich in starches, sugars, and fats and reduce intake of milk, meat, fish, fruits, and vegetables. Many poor elders are homeless or living in shelters, which may lack proper refrigeration and cooking facilities. Some poor seniors are getting enough calories in their diet and be of a normal weight or overweight. However, many of these non-underweight seniors are seriously lacking in many nutrients. While most seniors living in poverty are malnourished, it is important also to realize that a majority of seniors with adequate incomes are also malnourished.

Another factor affecting senior nutrition is the fact that many seniors do not drive a car and must rely on walking or help from others to obtain food. Many inner-city and rural elders do not have easy access to well-balanced diet. Food sources in many inner-city neighborhoods consist mostly of convenience stores, fast-food joints, and liquor shops and do not have easy access to supermarkets, restaurants, health food stores, fish, vegetable, and fruit markets (Inagami 2009). Such areas where healthy food is hard to obtain are called "food deserts". Other studies have also reported that getting little exercise and being housebound is associated with significantly poorer appetite and significantly poorer nutritional status (Sharkey 2008).

Drugs Worsen Appetite and Increase Nutrient Needs

Prescription drug use can also worsen nutrition. The median number of drugs that US adults is taking is three, with many seniors taking five to ten prescription drugs at a time (Minnesota Board of Aging 2002). Taking a number of medications at once can increase risk of nutritional problems by decreasing appetite and/or depleting the body of nutrients. Many prescription drugs can reduce appetite in seniors, including many antibiotics such as erythromycin, stimulants like Adderall, Lupron (used to treat prostate cancer), narcotics like OxyContin, antiseizure drugs like Topomax and Depakote, antidepressants like Prozac and Zoloft, and many other drugs (eMed Expert 2009).

In addition to reducing appetite, many prescription drugs also deplete the body of many nutrients. For example, many drugs can lower the blood and tissue levels of coenzyme Q_{10}, a vitamin-like substance important in the production of energy and in detoxification reactions. Common drugs, which lower coenzyme Q_{10} levels, include the cholesterol-lowering statins (Lipitor, Pravachol, Zocor); thiazide medications to lower blood pressure (Diuril); beta-blocker drugs (Lopressor); antidiabetic drugs (Glucotrol); and tricyclic antidepressants (Elavil) (University of Maryland 2005). Use of antiulcer drugs such as the H2 receptor antagonists (Pepcid) can reduce intestinal absorption and decrease the body's levels of many important nutrients such as vitamins B_{12}, C, and D and folate and minerals such as calcium, iron, and zinc (Pelton 2009). Aspirin reduces the body's uptake of vitamin C (Johnson2002). Many diuretics reduce the body's stores of many B vitamins and minerals such as potassium, magnesium, and calcium (Johnson 2002). The anticholesterol drug Questran and many antibiotics deplete the body of the fat soluble vitamins A, D, and E (Johnson 2002). Many other common prescription drugs can also deplete the body of a wide range of nutrients.

Empty Calories, Meal Skipping and Alcohol Reduce Nutritional Intakes

Consumption of high amounts of "empty calories" in the form of refined sugars (sugar, corn syrup, honey, etc.) and refined grains (such as white flour and white rice) can also increase risk of elder malnutrition. Refined sugars and grains contain many calories, but provide few nutrients and displace more nutritious foods like meat, fish, low-fat dairy, fruit, vegetables, and whole grains. Whole grain products are much more nutritious since they contain the germ and the bran where most of the fiber, vitamins, and minerals from the grain are found. The author remembers that all four of his grandparents were very fond of sweets like cakes, pies, cookies, and ice cream. One of his grandmothers frequently said, "I would be happy to live on nothing but deserts". A nationwide US survey reported that the average adult over age 60 years consumes about 64 pounds of added sugars (sugar, corn syrup, maple syrup, honey, etc.), which comprises about 17% of their calorie intake (Thompson 2009). In 2003, the average US adult consumed 10 servings of grain products daily, but only 1.5 of these servings were whole grain products (Mancino 2005).

Skipping meals, especially breakfast, has shown to be associated with significantly lowered nutritional intake. While elders are more likely to eat breakfast than younger adults, still about 8-18% of adults over 70 regularly skip breakfast (Song 2006). Skipping breakfast in the elderly has been associated with significant higher rates of heart disease, poorer blood sugar control in diabetics, lower levels of energy, and higher death rates (Timlin 2007).

Heavy alcohol consumption can also greatly increase risk of elder malnutrition. Roughly 6% of all seniors consume more than two alcoholic drinks per day, and perhaps 2% are full-blown alcoholics (Rigler 2000). In many cases, the alcohol problems of seniors are well hidden from friends and family. About one-third of all elderly alcoholics did not have a drinking problem in earlier life, but developed one later on due to various factors such as medical problems or loss of spouse, friends, and jobs. Alcoholic beverages have many empty calories but few nutrients. Alcoholics are often low in many nutrients including protein, magnesium, calcium, zinc, and many vitamins—especially thiamine (B_1), folate, vitamin B_{12}, and vitamin C (Auerhahn 1992).

Poorer Absorbtion of Nutrients in Elders

Another reason why elderly people are at a high risk of nutritional problems is that they do not absorb many nutrients as well as they did when they were younger. For example, vitamin B_{12} deficiency is found in as many as 40.5% of all elderly folks over age 70 years (Lindenbaum 1994). Vitamin B_{12} from foods that enters the stomach are in binds to a molecule called the "intrinsic factor". The intrinsic factor assists vitamin B_{12} absorption in the intestines. In many people over age 70 years, the production of intrinsic factors ceases or becomes greatly diminished. Loss of the intrinsic factor and other problems with digestive malabsorption such as decay of the lining of the intestinal cavity (atrophic gastritis) cause many elders to be vitamin B_{12} deficient even if they are consuming the Recommended Daily Allowance (RDA) of B_{12} in their diets (Andres 2005; Wolters 2004)

Lack of Sunlight Creates Vitamin D Deficiency

Lack of sunlight also plays a role in the vitamin D deficiencies seen in over 76% of seniors. Many seniors use sunblock when in the sun or are housebound and get little sun exposure. Sunblock can reduce risk of cancer but also increase risk of vitamin D deficiency unless sufficient vitamin D is given in the diet (Stechschulte 2009).

Illness and Depression Worsen Nutrition

Chronic and acute illnesses often found in the elderly can also greatly increase nutrition problems by limiting appetite and increase need for nutrients. For example many types of cancer and many infections greatly reduce appetite and also greatly increase the body's need for protein, calories, omega-3 and 6 fatty acids, and many vitamins and minerals (Van Cutsem 2005; Fearon 2008; Campbell 1999; Wintergerst 2007). Thus, patients with cancer and/or infections suffer a "double whammy" nutritionally, since appetite is often suppressed at a time nutritional needs are increased. Many illnesses such as Alzheimer's disease and Parkinson's disease can also greatly decrease appetite and also decrease the ability of the patient to feed themselves (Smith 2008).

Depression and bereavement can also cause weight loss and malnutrition. Death of a spouse often causes the surviving spouse to lose significant amounts of weight in months following the death (Schulz 2001). Other studies have noted that consumption of fruits vegetables, meat, fish, low-fat dairy products, and other healthy foods often declines following widowhood (Quandt 2000). In some cases, the spouse that died was the spouse who bought and prepared all of the family food. The surviving spouse may have to learn some shopping and cooking skills.

Malnutrition is Usually not Recognized or Documented by Physicians

Elders often enter hospitals in a malnourished condition (Kubrak and Jensen 2007). Seniors are often kept for days following surgery or other medical procedures without any nutrition at all or at most an intravenous (IV) solution containing only water, sugar, sodium, and potassium salts. This is called NPO, or *nil per os* (nothing by mouth). During medical school, The author was surprised at the number of patients kept NPO for five or more days. Poor hospital nutrition can greatly increase risk of infection, poor wound healing, and death, while good nutrition can speed recovery and prevent many deaths. Chapter 7 of this book will discuss hospital nutrition in detail.

Most US medical schools provide little training in nutrition, and what little training is offered is rarely given in a specific nutrition course but given as bits and pieces in other courses like biochemistry and physiology. A survey of 106 of the 126 US medical schools in 2004 reported that the average medical student received only twenty-three hours of nutrition instruction (Adams 2004). This is less than half of them time spent in a standard introductory nutrition class. This lack of nutritional training means that most physicians are poor at diagnosing and treating malnutrition in the elderly. The late noted Harvard nutrition professor Jean Mayer, PhD, pointed out that "the average physician knows about as much about nutrition as his secretary, unless the secretary belongs to Weight Watchers, in which case the secretary knows twice as much" (Crook1986).

While malnutrition is present in 42-91% of hospitalized seniors, their malnutrition usually goes unreported, untreated, and unnoticed (Kubrak and Jensen 2007). A nutritional study of 23,164 hospitalized patients older than 65 years in Ontario in 2000 reported that about 60% of these patients were malnourished, but less than 1 in 1,000 malnourished patients was given a diagnosis of malnutrition either orally or in their medical charts (Bobcock 2009).

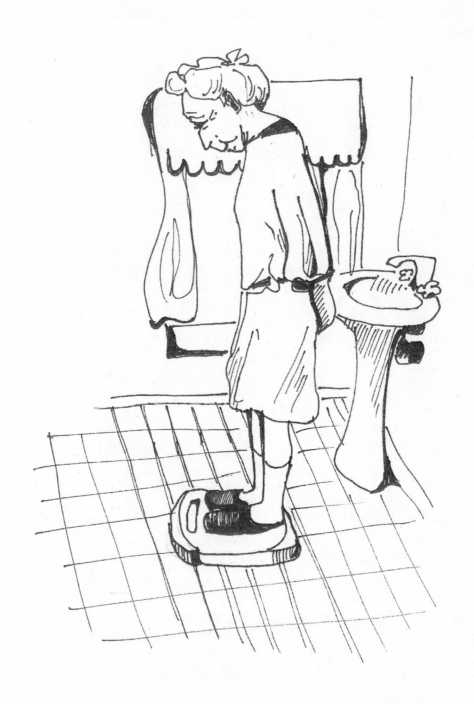

CHAPTER 3

WEIGHT CONCERNS: IN SENIORS, OVERWEIGHT IS SOMETIMES A PROBLEM, BUT UNDERWEIGHT A MORE COMMON AND OFTENTIMES A WORSE PROBLEM

M uch attention has been focused in recent years on the increase in overweight in the USA.

The number of heavy people in the USA has grown rapidly in the past twenty years. For example, in 1990 only 13% of the adult USA population was considered to be obese, while by 2005, that number had doubled to about 26% (CDC 2009). Those with a body mass index (BMI) of over 30 are considered obese (please see below for explanation of BMI). About 6% of US adults are severely or morbidly obese (BMI of 40).

Measuring Underweight and Overweight

Obesity can be measured a number of ways. The most common way to determine obesity is the body mass index or BMI. Body mass in kilograms (1 kilogram = 2.2 pounds) is divided by the square of a person's height in meters (1 meter = 39.3 inches). A "normal" BMI is from 18.5 to 25. A BMI of below 18.5 is considered underweight, a BMI between 25 and 30 is considered overweight, 30 to 35 is called mildly obese, 35 to 40 moderately obese, and over 40 is considered seriously or morbidly obese. To calculate BMI from height in pounds and height in feet and inches please see the following table below. To determine what BMI category a person of a certain height and weight would fall into, please see the table below. To calculate your BMI precisely, please see http://www.nhlbisupport.com/bmi/. Remember that a person with a large bone or muscle structure can have a fairly high BMI and still be quite lean.

Table to Calculate Body Mass Index Range (BMI or body mass index in kilograms/meters in height squared) from Height (in feet and inches) and Weight in Pounds							
	BODY MASS INDEX						
	Under-weight BMI less than 19	Normal Weight 19 to 25	Over-weight 26 to 30	Mild Obesity 31 to 35	Moderate Obesity 36 to 40	Morbid Obesity 41 to 50	Severe Obesity 50 plus
Height In Feet and Inches	BODY WEIGHT IN POUNDS						
4'10"	Under 91	91-119	120-143	144-167	168-191	192-239	240 +
4'11"	Under 94	94-124	125-148	149-173	174-198	199-247	247 +
5'0"	Under 97	98-128	129-153	154-179	180-204	205-255	256+
5'1"	Under 100	101-132	133-158	159-185	186-211	212-264	265+
5'2"	Under 104	105-136	137-164	165-191	192-218	219-273	274+
5'3"	Under 107	108-141	142-169	170-197	198-225	226-282	283 +
5'4"	Under 110	110-145	146-174	175-204	205-232	233-291	292 +
5'5"	Under 114	115-150	151-180	181-210	211-240	241- 300	300 +
5'6"	Under 118	119-155	156-186	187-216	217-247	248-309	310 +
5'7"	Under 121	122-159	160- 191	192-223	224-255	256-319	320 +
5'8"	Under 125	126-164	165-197	198-230	231-262	263-328	329 +
5'9"	Under 128	128-169	170-203	204-236	237-270	271-338	339+
5'10"	Under 132	133-174	175-209	210-243	244-278	279-348	349+
5'11"	Under 136	137-179	180-215	216-250	251-286	287-358	359+
6'0"	Under 140	141-184	185-221	222-258	259-294	295--368	369+
6'1"	Under 144	145-189	190-227	228-265	266-302	303- 378	379+
6'2"	Under 148	149-194	195-233	234-272	273-311	312-389	390+
6'3"	Under 152	153-200	201-240	241-279	280-319	320-399	400+
6'4"	Under 156	157-205	206-246	247-287	288-328	329-410	411+

LUKE CURTIS, MD

A more accurate way of determining obesity or excessive fat is to determine body fat percentage. Body fat can be determined in a number of ways including by measuring skin fat thickness and by weighing a person in water. Men should aim for 10-25% total body fat; women should be in the 15-30% range.

Relying too much on BMI indexes instead of fat percentages can produce unusual results. For example, muscular people can be in the overweight or mildly obese category and still be quite lean. In 2004, both candidates for US president, George Bush and John Kerry, were in the overweight category, yet both were physically active and appeared quite lean, with low body fat percentages.

Obesity increases risk of many chronic diseases like heart disease, stroke, diabetes, eye problems, some forms of cancer, sleep apnea, depression, and joint problems (Berke, 2000).

Why are Obesity Rates on the Rise?

Why the recent rise in obesity in the USA? While genetics plays some role in obesity, the biggest reason for the recent obesity surge is the current environment, which discourages exercise and encourages consumption of diets rich in fat and refined sugars. The per person consumption of sugars (including cane/beet sugar and corn syrup) in the United States is now over 142 pounds per year, up 19% since 1970 (US Department of Agriculture 2007). Many of these added sugars are found in soft drinks, sports drinks, heavily sweetened coffee, and other beverages. Restaurant meals are also getting larger. For example, the McDonald's Value Meal of a Big Mac hamburger, large fries and large Coke provides 1,350 calories, which is a lot of calories for a person who is not physically active. (McDonald's 2009).

Physical activity has also been reduced in recent years as fewer people have physically demanding jobs and fewer people walk or bicycle to school, work, shopping, or worship. The physical environment of many new towns and suburbs discourages walking and bicycling. Many new housing developments have no sidewalks or streetlights and funnel traffic into high-speed, high traffic-arterial roads, which discourage walking and bicycling.

With Age, Obesity Rates Decline and Underweight Increases

While overweight is a serious health problem in many adults and some seniors, the prevalence of obesity greatly declines past age 70 and rates of underweight greatly increase. A 2003 US Centers for Disease Control (CDC) survey reported US obesity rates of 26% among those aged 50 to 69 years, but only 16% among those older than 70 years (Center on an Aging Society 2009). A study of 23.8 million Canadian adults reported that the rates of severe underweight (BMI below 18.5) was only 0.7% among adults aged 55 to 64 years, but rose to 1.9% of adults aged 65 to 74 years and 4.2% of those over age 75 (Statistics Canada 2003). This same study also reported that overweight and obesity fell substantially after age 75. Overweight (BMI 25-30) and obesity (BMI 30+) respectively were 39.4% and 20.0% from age 55 to 64, 40.2% and 17.0% at age 65 to 74 years, and 35.1% and 10.9% for those over 75 years (Statistics Canada 2003).

Many studies have reported that elders in the underweight BMI category or even in the "normal" BMI group have more health problems and higher death rates than seniors in the "overweight" group. Underweight places elderly people at greater risk for many illnesses such as infectious diseases, bone loss (osteoporosis), and muscle loss (sarcopenia) (Schneider 2004; Asomaning 2006; Lee 2007). Research has indicated that seniors aged 65 to 80 years in the "overweight" BMI category have death rates and the life expectancy equal to or slightly lower than those in the "normal weight" (Jannsen 2007). Among seniors older than 80 years old, some studies have reported significantly lower mortality rates among those in the overweight group versus the normal weight groups (Corrada 2006). A study of death rates in 3,110 elderly Italians reported that death rates were lowest in the BMI group of 26-28, which corresponds to the overweight group. Compared to the BMI group of 26-28, elders with a BMI below 20 had 2.9 times as high a death rate, and those with a BMI of 20-22 (the middle of the "normal" weight group) had a mortality rate 1.6 times as great (results very statistically significant). Among elders with a body mass index of 30-34 (mildly obese), death rates were only 1.05 times as high as in the BMI group of 26-28 (Sergi 2005).

A number of studies have reported that significant weight loss in seniors who are not obese is associated with higher rates of illness, lower quality of life, and higher death rates (Leon-Munoz 2005). Weight loss in seniors with cancer is associated with higher illness and death rates in seniors. For example, a study of 3,047 cancer patients found that survival time in patients with 5% or more weight loss was significantly shorter in nine out of twelve chemotherapy protocols (Dewys 1980). This same study reported that among 290 patients with favorable non-Hodgkins lymphoma, five-year survival rates were 90% among 199 patients who had not lost more than 5% of their weight, but only 33% among 91 patients who lost more than 5% of their prelymphoma weight (results statistically very significant) (Dewys 1980).

During the author's thousands of hour of work in elder care facilities, he has noticed that many of the fairly healthy residents older than 85 years are a bit "chubby". Rapid weight loss in this age group is often a signal of impeding severe illness or death.

Avoiding Excess Water Retention

Many malnourished elders may appear too fat due to excess water retention or edema. Excess water often collects in the feet, lower legs, abdomen, and hands. The excess water retention is usually due to one of two factors: heart problems or low levels of the protein albumin of the blood. Albumin is a protein in the blood that plays a crucial role in transporting many nutrients and in maintaining water balance in the blood and tissue. Normal levels of albumin in the blood are from 3 to 5% (or 3.0 to 5.0 grams per 100 milliliters of blood). Albumin levels often become low in elders who have a poor diet and do not consume enough protein. Such low albumin levels cause fluid to leave the blood and collect in body tissues, causing edema and often giving feet, legs, and hands a "water-logged" appearance. Low levels of albumin in blood have been linked to higher levels of infection and heart disease.

While albumin levels are often low in the elderly, providing a better diet usually improves blood albumin levels and eliminates edema. A study of nineteen adults aged 63 to 79 years reported that feeding them diets fairly high in protein for twelve days significantly increased both body synthesis and blood levels of albumin. Subjects were given diets containing 1.0 gram of protein per kilogram of body weight daily, which is equal to 70 grams of protein for a 70-kilogram (154-pound) person (Thalacker-Mercer 2007).

All elders should consume a good source of protein at every meal at least three times daily. Most authorities suggest elders consume at least 60-80 grams of high-quality protein daily. A 3-to-4-ounce serving of lean meat or fish has about 15-20 grams of protein. A cup of milk/yogurt or an ounce of hard cheese has about 8 grams of protein, while half a cup of cottage cheese has 14 grams of protein. Two eggs contain 12 grams of very high-quality protein. Nuts, seeds, beans, and whole grain breads and cereals also contain modest about of protein. For a table of protein content in common foods, please see the protein section in chapter 18.

How Heavy Elders Can Lose Weight

What should elders do when they feel they are overweight and need to lose a few pounds?

They should first consult a physician and get their fat content determined. If their fat percentage is less than 25% for men or 30% for women, they probably do not need to lose weight. Many seniors who appear a little overweight are really just a bit flabby. Regular exercise can often give them a firmer, tighter appearance without losing any weight.

Some elders do need to lose some weight. The best ways of losing weight for elderly seem to involve a combination of a well-balanced diet with adequate fiber and protein at every meal and exercise for at least thirty minutes at least three times weekly (McTigue 2006). Elders should plan to lose about 1 pound per week; faster weight loss programs are dangerous and often cause loss of lean muscle mass as well as fat. Empty calories such as refined sugar, corn syrup, saturated fats (fat from meats, dairy products and fats from processed foods like margarine and potato chips) and refined grains (like white rice and white flour) should be avoided. Eating breakfast every day and consuming at least five servings of fruits and vegetables daily are also associated with lower body weight and fat levels (Raynor 2008; He 2004). Most fruits and vegetables are ideal for weight control diets since they are high in fiber and nutrients and low in calories unless they are prepared with added sugar or fat.

Generally speaking, the most effective weight loss regimes involve both exercise and improved diet. One particularly effective program involved overweight middle-aged or elderly men who ate a low-fat diet for three years. In addition to the low-fat diet, part of this group also was instructed to eat at least 1 pound of fruits and vegetables daily and exercise daily (such as brisk walking). In three years, the 210 men who exercised and ate the fruits and vegetables daily lost an average of 14 pounds, while the 232 men treated only with the low-fat diet lost an average of only 5 pounds. In addition, the men getting the daily exercise also had a significantly lower rate of heart attacks, significant drops in blood pressure and LDL ("bad") cholesterol and significantly improved blood sugar control as compared to the men receiving only the low-fat diet intervention (Singh 1996).

Losing excess weight is difficult at any age. Studies of many weight loss plans report that average weight loss in a year is only about 5 to 10 pounds (Brown 2009). However, losing a modest amount of weight, such as 10 pounds in a moderately overweight senior, can greatly alleviate many overweight-related health problems such as diabetes, heart disease, high blood pressure, arthritis/joint problems, and sleep apnea (Web MD 2009).

Involvement of weight loss groups such as Weight Watchers or Jenny Craig also can be useful for many seniors. Some of these weight loss centers have special programs for seniors. Exercise is also often more effective in groups. Elders needing to lose weight should consider joining a fitness, water exercise, or dance class or joining a walking, bicycling, or tennis club.

Many good diet books are also available to help in losing weight. Look for a well-balanced diet, which emphasizes fruits, vegetables, fish, and low-fat meats and dairy products. The diet should also avoid sugars, refined grains, and saturated and trans fats. One of the author's favorite diet books is *The South Beach Diet* (Agatston 2004). The South Beach Diet emphasizes lean meat, fish, nuts, fruits, and vegetables. Many of the author's larger patients have lost at least a few pounds on the South Beach Diet.

A number of good diet and cookbooks are available, which promote the Mediterranean Diet (Cloutier 2004). The Mediterranean Diet emphasizes fish, fruits, vegetables, whole grains, and olive oil. The author has also seen many chubby elders lose weight on this type of diet as well.

Gaining Weight Helpful for Underweight Seniors

Many seniors need to gain weight. Such elders should also consume at least three well-balanced meals with protein at every meal. High-calorie, high-protein foods like nuts, seeds, and cheese should be eaten daily. Underweight seniors also often benefit by consuming a nutritional drink like Boost or Ensure daily. Chapter 17 and many of the following chapters give many suggestions for a well-balanced diet, which can maintain a healthy weight for seniors. Seniors who remain underweight in spite of a good diet should consult their physician to rule out non-nutritional causes of overweight such as overactive thyroid gland (hyperthyroid), cancer, intestinal parasites, or intestinal malabsorption.

Later chapters of this book will discuss specific health problems related to elder malnutrition. The later chapters will also give recommendations about how to improve the diets and provide adequate food supplements for seniors. Such nutritional improvements can prevent or mitigate common chronic health problems. Many foods and nutrients are important in preventing or alleviating many types of health problems. For example, consuming five or more servings daily of a wide range of fruits and vegetables can help prevent heart disease, strokes, high blood pressure, overweight, eye problems, and many types of cancer.

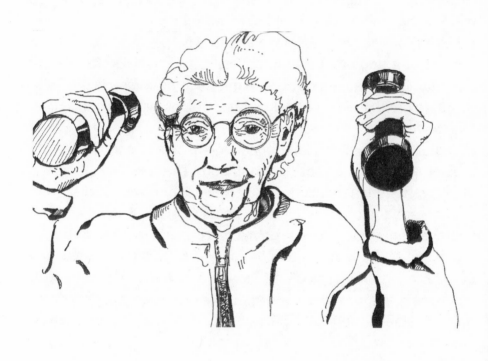

CHAPTER 4

NUTRITION AND EXERCISE FOR TREATING MUSCLE LOSS (SARCOPENIA)

Muscle Loss Is a Common and Debilitating Problem in Elders that Gets Little Media Attention

M uscle loss is a major problem for many elderly people. The technical term for muscle loss is "sarcopenia". Many older folks start to experience loss of muscle mass in their fifties and sixties. Studies have shown that an adult's average muscle weight tends to decline at a rate of about 1% per year after age 50 years, with declines being greater in men and sedentary elders as compared to women and active elders (Hughes 2002). By the seventies, many seniors have lost a significant percentage of muscle on their arms, legs, abdomen, chest, shoulder, hands, feet, and head/face. Some seniors show noticeable wasting of muscles on the face, arms, and legs. Their skin often sags a great deal due to loss of muscle mass. A US survey of 4,449 adults older than 60 years reported that 31.3% of the women and 64.3% of the men had moderate to severe sarcopenia (Jannsen 2004). A New Mexico survey reported that in adults over 80, about 50% of men and 40% of women have significant sarcopenia (Baumgartner 1998).

While muscle loss (sarcopenia) has received much less attention in the popular press and media than bone loss (osteoporosis), the effects of sarcopenia can be just as devastating. Major loss of muscle can limit mobility and activities like walking and feeding, increase risk of physical disability, slow wound healing, and increase risk for falls and other accidents and illnesses (Jannsen 2004; Zacker 2006). Such loss of lean muscle mass reduces breathing and exercise capacity and significantly increases risk for infection and death (Thomas 2007; Cosqueric 2006; Cawthon 2006). Large amounts of muscle loss can even occur among overweight or obese elderly people, a condition called "sarcopenic obesity" (Zamboni 2008).

A Well-Balanced Diet and Exercise Are Crucial for Building and Maintaining Muscle Mass

How can sarcopenia be prevented or even partially reversed? The cornerstones of preventing muscle loss or regaining lost muscle are a good diet and sufficient exercise. Many studies have reported that some of the muscle lost due to a sarcopenia can be regained by a well-balanced diet sufficient in protein and calories along with adequate exercise. Human and animal studies have found that consumption of a well-balanced diet with many nutrients is helpful in preventing or regaining lost muscle mass. Some of these nutrients include (Siddiqui 2006; Semba 2007; Kim 2010) the following:

1) Calories: Sufficient calories are essential as muscle building is difficult without sufficient energy.
2) Sufficient amino acids from proteins, especially good protein sources include milk (including whey protein supplements), eggs, meats, and fish. Elders with muscle

loss should consume at least 1.2 to 1.5 grams of protein per kilogram of bodyweight (or 0.6 to 0.7 grams per pound of bodyweight). A 100 pound elder with muscle loss should consume at least 60 to 70 grams of protein daily. A 4-ounce serving of lean meat and fish has 14-20 grams of protein, a cup of milk/yogurt, or an ounce of cheese has about 8 grams, and 2 eggs have 12 grams of protein. Whole grains, soybeans, peanuts, and other beans also provide some protein. For a more complete table of protein in common foods, please see the protein section in chapter 18.

3) The amino acids creatine, glutamine, arginine, leucine, and beta-hydroxy-beta-methylbutyrate (a leucine derivative) may be especially helpful in regaining lost muscle mass.

4) Omega-3 fatty acids have been shown in many studies to be helpful in reversing sarcopenia. Omega-3 fats are found in fish oil; fatty fish (such as salmon, herring, anchovies, sardines, and mackerel); and flax oil. Lesser amounts of omega-3 fats are found in soybean and canola oils, walnuts, and pumpkin seeds. Much more about the health effects of omega-3 fats will be mentioned in following chapters. For more information about sources of omega-3 fats, please see omega-3 fats section in chapter 18.

5) Conjugated linolenic acid, which is a fatty acid found in beef and milk fats. The author recommends consuming beef, milk, or cheese daily to get valuable conjugated linolenic acid.

6) Carotenoids, which are a form of vitamin A found in yellow fruits and vegetables.

7) Vitamin D helps in preventing sarcopenia. Vitamin D is found in supplements, vitamin D-fortified milk, eggs, and fatty fish. Vitamin D can also be produced by skin exposed to sunlight. Analysis of five published studies have reported that elders supplied with 400 to 800 international units daily of supplemental vitamin D had significantly

less muscle wasting and an average of 22% fewer falls than those not given supplemental vitamin D (Bischoff 2004). Retaining or regaining muscle mass and strength is believed to be very helpful in preventing falls in seniors.

8) Polyphenols are helpful in reversing sarcopenia. Polyphenols are "phytochemicals" found in a wide range of fruits and vegetables. Five servings (half a cup of more) of a wide range of fruits and vegetables daily should provide elders with sufficient polyphenols.

It is important that elders eat at least three well-balanced meals daily containing sufficient protein. A high-protein breakfast, which includes milk, yogurt, eggs, cottage cheese, low-fat meats, fish, or soy products is a great way to maintain muscle mass and fight sarcopenia. High-protein foods like nuts, sunflower or pumpkin seeds, low-fat milk or cheese, fish, and low-fat meats also make great snacks. Three or more smaller meals throughout the day is better for maintaining energy levels and muscle mass than one or two large meals late in the day. As noted in chapter 2, many elders do not consume sufficient protein or calories in a day to maintain muscle mass. A number of published studies have reported that eating three or more meals a day consisting of at least 25 grams of protein in each meal are useful in maintaining muscle mass and preventing sarcopenia (Paddon-Jones 2009). For a table of protein content in common foods, please see the protein section in chapter 18.

A particularly useful protein supplement for sarcopenic patients is whey protein isolate. Whey protein isolate is obtained from the liquid portion of milk (whey) after the curds have been removed to make cheese. Whey protein has an excellent balance of amino acids and has been shown to be well absorbed and stimulates protein synthesis in the elderly (Hayes 2008). Whey protein is available at reasonable cost from many supplement and health food stores. Several studies have shown that protein supplementation with whey or milk protein can significantly increase muscle mass in seniors with muscle loss (sarcopenia) (Kim 2010).

Another excellent amino acid supplement for regaining muscle loss in sarcopenic patients are mixtures of arginine, glutamine, and either leucine or beta-hydroxy-beta-methylbutyrate (a leucine derivative). These amino acids can be obtained at health food stores or compound pharmacies or obtained commercially in such products as Juven (Abbott Labs).

Use of these amino acid mixtures containing arginine, glutamine, and leucine can produce dramatic results in people with muscle wasting. For example, a double-blind study conducted with sarcopenic HIV patients reported that eight weeks' supplementation with arginine, glutamine, and HMB was associated with an average 2.55 kilogram (5.6 pound) gain in lean body mass while patients given placebo had a mean of 0.70 kilogram (1.5 pound) loss in lean body mass (results statistically very significant) (Clark 2000).

Consuming five or more servings of fruits and vegetables provide many vitamins, minerals, and phytochemicals necessary to maintain muscle mass. Eating fatty fish (such as salmon, mackerel, anchovies, sardines, and herring) several times a week not only provides a lot of excellent quality protein, but also provides considerable vitamin D and omega-3 fats. Cod-liver oil and fish oil are also very rich in both vitamin D and omega-3 fats. Sufficient protein, omega-3 fats, and vitamin D are all necessary for building and maintaining healthy muscle mass. As noted in chapter 2, the vast majority of elders are low in both vitamin D and omega-3 fats.

Exercise Regularly at Activities You Enjoy

A modest amount of weight lifting, stationary bike riding, and treadmill walking has been shown to significantly increase muscle mass, strength, and improve cardiovascular fitness in frail people those over 80 years (Fiatarone 1990; Vaitkevincius 2002). One study found that moderate exercise could almost triple strength in the quadricep muscles (found in the front part of the thigh) in adults over age 90 years! (Fiatarone 1990). Another study had twenty-five adults older than 70 years participate in a weight lifting program twice a week. These older athletes did a series of weight lifting exercises including leg press, chest (bench) press, leg extension, leg flexion, shoulder press, lat pull down, seated row, calf raise, abdominal crunch, and back extension. Following twenty-six weeks of weight lifting exercises, the average muscle strength of the twenty-five old athletes increased by an average of 50%! (Melov 2007). In addition, biochemical and genetic studies of the older athletes reported that the regular weight lifting significantly increase the body's production of proteins to levels more typically seen in younger people (Melov 2007).

It is important to pick an exercise activity you enjoy so you will stick with exercising over the long haul. Walking, bicycling, swimming, golf, tennis, table tennis, weight lifting, gardening, dancing, exercise class, and active play with grandchildren are all common forms of exercise that seniors enjoy. Use of indoor stationary bicycles are especially useful for people with balance problems or for use during bad weather. Veteran athletes also frequently use a variety of weight machines to maintain strength in a wide range of muscles. Use of free weights are also useful, but many require the use of a spotter to prevent the athlete from dropping the weight (Taaffe 2006). Outdoor exercise in sunny weather also provides the benefit of vitamin D from sunlight. However, prolonged exposure to sunlight when the sun is above 30 degrees from the horizon may cause burning, especially in fair-skinned people. Sunblock may be needed for exposure to the sun lasting more than thirty minutes.

The author knows of many seniors over the age of 80 who regularly walk, bike, swim, golf, play tennis, and lift weights.

LUKE CURTIS, MD

The author knows a 78-year-old woman who regularly leads an exercise class at a local fitness center.

Working with an exercise partner or group is also helpful in enabling many people to stick to an exercise regime. Many fitness clubs, YM(W)C(H)As, community recreation facilities, and senior centers have exercise programs or groups specifically for "veteran" athletes. Many fitness facilities also have coaches and personal trainers who are delighted to show novices the proper use of exercise equipment or the proper form for dance exercise or calisthenics. Some programs are designed for seniors with specific health challenges, such as water exercise classes for those with joint problems and medically supervised programs for those with heart conditions. Consulting a physical therapist can also be useful in recommending a specific exercise regime for elders with various muscle and joint injuries. The author encourages all seniors to look for exercise opportunities in their communities.

Proper diet and exercise can often greatly build back muscle mass dramatically in people in their eighties and nineties. The author knows of a gentleman who was confined to a wheelchair after losing a lot of muscle following surgery at age 82. The muscles on his arms and face were so thin that they were hard to look at. The fellow was quite depressed and ready to give up on life. However, the author suggested he improve his diet and undergo physical therapy. He improved his diet by eating lots of meat, fish, fruits, vegetables, whole grains, and low-fat dairy products. He supplemented his diet with a good multivitamin mineral supplement, whey protein, and 4 one gram capsules of fish oil daily. He also drank a can or two a nutritional supplement drink like Boost or Ensure. At the author's suggestion, he underwent an aggressive period of physical therapy. He gradually gained strength, and at 84, he is walking well with a cane. This gentleman has gained about 20 pounds, and his muscles look much fuller and stronger. He is also going to the local fitness club regularly to ride a bike and lift weights—including bench-pressing 105 pounds! This fellow is now spending his time going to church and other activities with his wife, working on the library board, and tending to his grass and garden at home.

Good diet, proper supplements, and regular exercise are critical for maintaining both muscle and bone mass. The next chapter will focus on diet and exercise for maintaining bone mass.

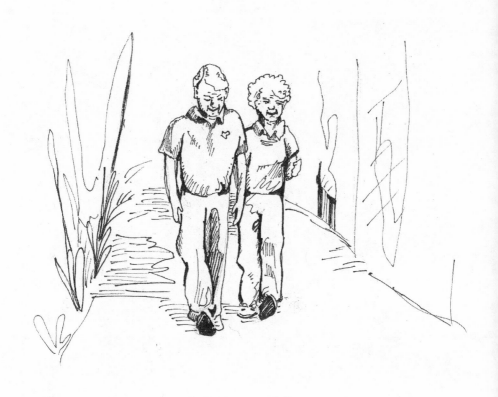

CHAPTER 5

NUTRITION AND EXERCISE FOR TREATING BONE LOSS (OSTEOPOROSIS)

Bone Loss Is Also Common and Debilitating in Seniors

Loss of bone mass or thinning of bones is often devastating to seniors. The technical term for this is "osteoporosis". About 8 million women and 2 million men over the age of 60 years have osteoporosis (Sweet 2009). About one in two US women can expect to experience an osteoporosis-related fracture in her lifetime. Osteoporosis is very common in all senior groups, but is most common in women, Caucasians, thin people, and people with a family history of osteoporosis. Osteoporosis greatly increases the risk of bones breaking after some minor trauma, like a mild fall. Sometimes, bones of patients with osteoporosis break for no apparent reason at all. Osteoporosis can also contribute to weak backbones and a poor, bent-over posture in elders.

Osteoporosis-related fractures have been shown to greatly reduce senior mobility and increase risk of infection and death (Sweet 2009). Hip fractures are often particularly debilitating, very painful and cause a great deal of mental depression and take months to heal. The average cost of treating a hip fracture is about $43,000, with 25% of all hip fracture patients requiring long-term nursing care (Sweet 2009). The author remembers his beloved maternal grandmother being debilitated for many months after breaking her hip at age 83 years.

Age-related changes in hormones can also increase risk of osteoporosis. Lack of estrogen can play a role in increasing risk of osteoporosis in postmenopausal women (Sweet 2009). Recent research has also found that lack of testosterone may play a role in osteoporosis in both men and women and that lack of estrogen may play a role in osteoporosis in men as well as women (Vandeput 2009). Patients with osteoporosis should discuss possible hormone treatments with their physicians.

Preventing Falls in Seniors

Since falls can easily cause bone breakage in osteoporosis patients, home prevention of falls is critical. Improved lighting of home, removing loose rugs, use of canes and walkers, and use of handrails near stairs, toilets, and bathtubs can reduce risk of falls in seniors. Since many medications can affect balance, all seniors with balance problems should have their medications evaluated by a physician to see if they are causing balance problems (Sweet 2009). The use of comfortable clothing and well-fitting and well-supportive shoes can also decrease risk of falls in elders with osteoporosis.

The diagnosis of osteoporosis is usually conducted by dual energy x-ray absorptiometry or a DEXA scan. DEXA is a painless procedure that is usually performed in physician's offices and often covered by health insurance. Many authorities recommend that all women age 65 years and all men over 70 years old receive a DEXA scan. Persons with severe thinning of the bones are diagnosed with osteoporosis, while less severe thinning of the bone is known as osteopenia.

LUKE CURTIS, MD

Seniors with thinning bones are often treated with a class of drugs called the bisphosphonates. The bisphosphonates include common drugs like Fosamax, Actonel, and Boniva. These drugs strengthen bone by reducing the loss of calcium in the bones. Several research studies have reported that use of bisphosphates significantly increases bone density and can significantly reduce risk of hip and back fractures (Sweet 2009). Estrogen supplements or the use of estrogen receptor modulators like Evista are sometimes helpful in treating postmenopausal women with thinning bones.

Nutrition can play a big role in preventing and treating osteoporosis. Physicians often recommend that their osteoporosis patients take supplements containing calcium and vitamin D. However, a comprehensive nutrition program and exercise can play a big role in preventing and treating osteoporosis, but is oftentimes overlooked. The remaining part of this chapter will discuss nutritional and exercise treatments for osteoporosis.

Need for Adequate Calcium, Vitamin D, Magnesium, and Other Nutrients to Maintain Bone

Many nutrients are needed to maintain and build healthy bones as we age. While many nutrients are needed for healthy bones, the two most important are probably calcium and vitamin D. Calcium comprises about 16% of bone mass, and vitamin D is critical for metabolic processes in which calcium from the blood is used to build bone. Calcium and vitamin D are usually very deficient in senior diets. Various studies have reported that the average US adult over age 60 years consumes only 20% of the USRDA for vitamin D and 60% of the USRDA for calcium (Park 2008). The USRDA for adults over 70 years are 1,200 milligrams daily of calcium and 400 international units of vitamin D (Whitney 2008).

Good dietary sources of calcium include milk, yogurt, cheese, and other dairy products, some green vegetables like broccoli and mustard greens, and fish eaten with bones, such as salmon, anchovies, and sardines. Sources of vitamin D in the diet are few and include vitamin D-supplemented milk, eggs, fatty fish like salmon, and fish oils like cod-liver oil (Whitney 2008). Vitamin D can also be produced in the skin by people exposed to sunlight; however, a majority of seniors do not get a lot of outdoor sun exposure.

Sufficient calcium and vitamin D are sometimes hard to get even in well-balanced diet. Many studies have reported that supplemental calcium and vitamin D can reduce risk of osteoporosis and bone fractures in the elderly. A meta-analysis of twenty-nine studies of 63,897 adults older than 50 years reported that consumption of 800 to 1,500 milligrams of calcium and 400 to 800 international units of vitamin D was associated with an overall, statistically significant 12% reduction in osteoporosis fractures (Tang 2007). Another meta-analysis of twenty studies with elders reported that daily supplementation of 700 to 1,100 international units daily associated with a statistically significant 23% drop in fractures, while only 400 international units a day was associated with no reduction in fracture risk (Bischoff 2009). Many of these studies also reported that bone density was significantly increased in elders consuming the calcium and vitamin D supplements (Tang 2007). Several studies have reported that taking 400 or more international units a day of vitamin D is associated with significantly less bone pain in osteoporosis patients (Stechshulte, 2009). The author recommends that all patients at risk for osteoporosis consume supplements containing at least 800 milligrams of calcium and 400 to 1,200 international units of vitamin D daily.

Strangely enough, some studies have reported that higher consumption of milk and dairy products has only a modest effect on reducing osteoporosis (Kanis 2005). Milk is high in both protein and calcium, and higher-protein diets require higher calcium levels since more calcium is lost in urine in people consuming higher protein diets.

While the use of calcium and vitamin D to prevent and treat osteoporosis has received most of the media attention, many other nutrients are also critical for healthy bone growth and maintenance. These nutrients include magnesium, vitamins K, C, and B complex, omega-3 fats, and phytochemicals such as carotenoids from yellow vegetables (like carrots) and soybean proteins.

Magnesium is a mineral involved in over five hundred chemical reactions in the body and plays a critical role in bone formation and in the control of bone metabolism hormones like parathyroid hormone. Magnesium is often deficient in US diets, with elderly women consuming on average only about 68% of the USRDA for magnesium (Rude 2009). Magnesium is found in a wide range of foods including nuts and seeds (especially pumpkin seeds), vegetables, whole grains, meats, and fish. Numerous human and animal studies have reported that low-magnesium diets can increase the risk of osteoporosis even if sufficient calcium and vitamin D are supplied (Rude 2009; Yaegashi 2008). Studies with young men have also reported that men given 360 milligrams of supplemental magnesium daily had significant less bone loss (Dimal 1998).

Other minerals can play a major role in building bone. Phosphorus comprises about 8% of bone. Most US adults receive adequate phosphorus in their diet, provided they are not deficient in calories and protein (Palacios 2006). Zinc is often deficient in elders and may play a role in osteoporosis. High-potassium intakes (over 4,700 milligrams a day) are associated with significantly lower rates of bone loss. Fruits and vegetables are high in potassium (especially potatoes, bananas, and citrus fruits like oranges and grapefruits). Several studies have reported high consumption of fruits and vegetables significantly increase bone density and reduce risk of osteoporosis-related fractures (Kitchin 2007). Consumption of the recommended five to ten one-half-cup servings of fruits and vegetables daily should provide adequate potassium for bone growth and many other body functions. High-fruit and vegetable consumption promote an alkaline environment in the body, which reduces loss of calcium from the bones (Palacious 2006).

Minor minerals like fluoride, copper, boron, selenium, and manganese also play an important role in bone growth (Palacious 2006). Fluoride is obtained through fluoridated water and toothpaste. Small amounts of fluoride are needed for bone and tooth growth while too much fluoride is harmful to bone and teeth. Copper, boron, selenium, and manganese are trace minerals often found in meats, fish, and in whole grains, fruits, vegetables. Many multimineral supplements contain small amounts of fluoride, copper, boron, and manganese.

Vitamin K is an important vitamin needed for blood clotting. Vitamin K is found in green and yellow vegetables and is also produced from other food by intestinal bacteria in the stomach. Several studies have reported that high consumption of vitamin K from vegetables and/or 1 milligram a day of supplemental vitamin K is associated with significantly less bone loss (Yaegashi 2008; Braam 2003).

Time for an important drug safety note: Green and yellow vitamin K-containing vegetables will partially reverse the effects of blood-thinning drugs like Coumadin used to reduce risk of blood clots in the body. Persons on blooding-thinning drugs like Coumadin should consume similar amounts of green and yellow leafy vegetables every day so that the doses of bone-thinning drugs can be adjusted accordingly. If persons on blood-thinning drugs consume green and yellow vegetables erratically, their blood will be too thick (too likely to clot) on days of high vegetable consumption and too thick (too thin to easily clot) on days of no vegetable consumption.

LUKE CURTIS, MD

Vitamin C is an important nutrient critical for formation of bone, muscle, skin, and gums and for maintaining immunity against disease. Vitamin C is found in many fruits and vegetables especially in oranges and grapefruit, cantaloupe, kiwi, tomatoes, broccoli, cabbage, strawberries, and potatoes. Several studies have reported that vitamin C consumption reduces risk of osteoporosis even in adults consuming adequate amounts of vitamin D and calcium. A study of 858 older US adults (average age of 75 years) reported that those who consumed more than 313 milligrams a day of vitamin C in the diet and supplements had a 44 % lower risk of hip fractures and a 34% lower risk of vertebral fractures (Sahni 2009).

Another study of 977 postmenopausal women reported that the women who consumed 500 or 1,000 milligrams of supplemental vitamin C daily had significantly higher bone mineral density than women who did not consume the vitamin C supplement (Morton 2001).

Other nutrients are useful in building or maintaining bone mass and strength. As mentioned in chapter 4, carotenoids from green and yellow vegetables are useful for preventing muscle wasting. A study of 946 elderly US adults reported that higher consumption of carotenoids were associated with significantly lower risk of hip fracture (Sahni 2009b). Lycopenes are red-colored phytochemicals produced by a number of fruits and vegetables including tomatoes, watermelon, and papaya. This same study of 946 US elderly adults also reported that higher lycopene consumption was associated with significantly lower rates of hip and nonvertebral fractures (i.e., nonback fractures) (Sahni 2009b). Soybeans contain proteins called isoflavones, which are somewhat similar in function to estrogen hormones. Some studies have reported that regular consumption of soybeans can reduce risk of osteoporosis and osteoporotic fractures (Ishimi 2009). A study of 95 elderly women with osteoporosis reported that supplementation with 6 grams (about 1.5 teaspoons) of fish oil and evening primrose oil daily resulted in significantly higher bone density and significantly lower rates of hip fracture (Kruger 1998). Human and animal studies have reported that regular consumption of plums and prunes are associated with significantly higher bone masses. The high levels of phenolic phytochemicals and the trace elements boron and selenium found in prunes and plums may be helpful to bone health (Hooshmand 2009).

Smoking, alcohol consumption, or heavy consumption of carbonated beverages like colas can also increase risk of bone loss (Kamel 2006). All patients in danger of osteoporosis should stop smoking and limit alcohol intake. Many smokers have quit successfully with the use of stop-smoking programs and/or the use of nicotine patches or gum. Nicotine patches and gum are available over the counter without a prescription in many states.

Strontium also Useful in Building Strong Bones

It is well known that a well-balanced diet and proper supplements containing sufficient calcium, phosphorus, magnesium, and vitamin D are needed to build and maintain strong bones over a lifetime. Less well known is that another mineral called strontium can also play a major role in building bone health. Strontium is a mineral that is on the same series of calcium on the periodic table of elements. Calcium is element number 20, while strontium is element number 38 and is sort of like a "big brother" or "big sister" to calcium. Strontium has many of the same properties of calcium, but it is heavier and denser than calcium. Small amounts of strontium are found in many foods such as vegetables, fruits, milk, and meat. Small quantities of strontium do not have any known adverse health effects, except for the radioactive form of strontium called strontium 90. Strontium 90 is highly radioactive and is produced from nuclear bomb explosions, while virtually all of the strontium found in foods and in food supplements is the nonradioactive form.

LUKE CURTIS, MD

A number of studies have reported that supplemental strontium is helpful in maintaining bone mass and preventing bone breakage in older patients at risk for osteoporosis. A French study gave 719 postmenopausal women with osteoporosis 2 grams (2,000 milligrams) of supplemental strontium ranelate daily, while 723 postmenopausal women with osteoporosis received placebo. All 1,441 women also received a supplement of 1,000 milligrams of calcium and 400 to 800 international units of vitamin D daily. The women were treated for three years with strontium or placebo. Following the three-year treatment, bone density in the vertebrae (back bones) increased by an average of 13% in the women receiving strontium but fell an average of 1% in the women given placebo. Bone density in the hip increased by an average of 8% in the women given the strontium supplement, while they fell an average of 2% in the women given placebo. The average rates of vertebrae (back) bones fractures were 41% less in the women given strontium, while rates of hip fracture were 10% lower in the women receiving strontium. There were no significant differences between with the two groups in terms of side effects such as diarrhea or headaches (Muenier 2005).

Strontium can be helpful in preventing fractures even in patients over 80 years of age. A study of 1,489 women over age 80 years was conducted over a five-year period in various clinics in Europe and Australia. As before, some women received a daily supplement of 2 grams strontium ranelate or placebo daily. All participants also received a supplement of vitamin D and calcium. Women taking the strontium supplement had a 31% lower risk of vertebrae fracture and 24% lower risk of hip fracture as compared to the women receiving placebo. As in the earlier strontium study, no increases in side effects were noted in the group given strontium as compared to placebo (Seeman 2009).

The author recommends that all persons with osteoporosis or at risk of osteoporosis consider adding 2 grams of strontium ranelate to their nutrition regime. Strontium ranelate is available without a prescription at health food and drug stores. In is important to realize that building bones is a fairly slow process and it may take several months to several years to build backbones that have been weakened by osteoporosis. It is also important to realize that many nutrients are required to build bone including protein, calcium, magnesium, boron, phosphorus, and many vitamins.

Exercise Critical in Maintaining and Building Healthy Bone Mass

Regular weight bearing exercise is critical for maintaining or even gaining bone mass in elders. About twelve published studies have reported that exercises like fast walking, treadmill walking, or weights can increase bone mass or at least prevent bone loss in those over sixty years (Guadalupe-Grau 2009). A few studies have also reported that postmenopausal women who exercise regularly have significantly lower rates of hip and back fractures (Walker 2000).

Lifetime exercise is also critical. Some studies have also reported that older adults who got large amounts of exercise during their teen and early adult years had significantly denser bones and significantly lower risk of bone fractures in old age (Guadalupe-Grau 2009).

Walking, weight lifting, tennis, golf (no motorized carts), and dancing are all excellent weight bearing exercises. Some good forms of exercise such as bicycling and swimming do not offer a high enough level of weight bearing to help build bone. As mentioned in chapter 4, it is important to pick a form of exercise that one enjoys so one will stick with the exercise.

As is the case with severe muscle loss, the author has seen many patients improve dramatically with a good diet and exercise. He knows of one 80-year-old lady who had broken both of her hips, several or her back bones (vertebrae), and her collarbone (scapula) over a several year period. These bone breaks have confined her largely to her home; she could no longer drive and could walk only with a walker. She was scared that she would break more bones. She had a bone DEXA scan, which indicated severe osteoporosis. At the author's suggestion, she improved her diet and ate mostly meat, fish, whole grains, fruits, vegetables, and low-fat dairy products. She also had a number of supplements daily including a general multivitamin/mineral tablet, plus four 1 gram capsules of fish oil, 1,000 milligrams of calcium, 500 milligrams of magnesium, 2,000 milligrams of strontium, and 1,000 international units of vitamin D daily. She got physical therapy and joined a water exercise class. At age 83, she now exercises by swimming half mile a day and/or attending a water exercise class. She also frequently walks 1 to 2 miles. Her back posture has improved significantly, and her bone DEXA scan is now almost at normal levels. Recently, this woman was well enough to drive 300 miles by herself to visit grandchildren in another state!

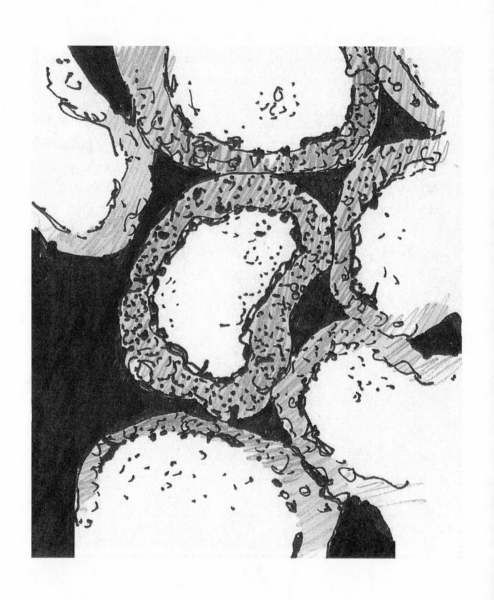

CHAPTER 6

NUTRITION TO PREVENT
AND TREAT INFECTION

T he recent concern about the H1N1 swine flu, development of bacteria resistant to multiple types of antibiotics, and the rise rates of hospital-acquired infections such as MRSA (methicillin-resistant *Staphylococcus aureus*) have focused public attention on avoiding infections. Due to tremendous overuse of antibiotics in both human health care and in raising farm animals, many bad infectious bacteria have developed resistance to a large number of antibiotics.

In spite of modern antibiotic treatment, several billion infections occur annually in the USA and many infections become fatal. In 2006, pneumonia and influenza (flu) killed an estimated 56,247 in the United States alone (CIDRAP 2008). Hospital-acquired infections are caused by a wide variety of bacteria, molds, and viruses and kill about 100,000 annually in the United States (Curtis 2008). Much more will be said about avoiding hospital-acquired infections in the following chapter (chapter 7) on hospital nutrition.

Nutrition Plays a Central Role in Fighting Infection

Nutrition plays a key role in maintaining the body's resistance to infection. Many nutrients play a key role in maintaining immunity including protein; omega-3 fatty acids; vitamins A, B_6, B_{12}, C, D, and E; selenium; zinc; copper; and iron (Wintergerst 2007). Most of these nutrients become depleted following chronic illness (Wintergerst 2007). Malnutrition is a major risk factor for infection. A French study of 630 hospitalized patients reported that the risk of hospital-acquired infections was five times as great in severely malnourished patients compared with adequately nourished patients (Schneider 2004). Other studies have reported that malnourished elderly (living at home, in an elder care facility, or in the hospital) are significantly more likely to acquire infections such as pneumonia compared with well-nourished elderly (Paillaud 2005; Rothan-Tondeur 2003).

Malnutrition in either children or adults greatly increases risks that common infections become fatal. In many developing countries, many common childhood infections often become fatal to malnourished children. For example, measles infections are now fatal to less than 1 in 10,000 children in the developed world, but measles fatality rates are as high as 20-40% has been reported among malnourished children in the developing world. It has been estimated that childhood malnutrition causes 1,000,000 additional deaths due to pneumonia, 800,000 more deaths from diarrhea, 500,000 more malaria deaths, and 250,000 more measles deaths as would have occurred if all children were well nourished (Caulfield 2004). It is tragic that many of these childhood infection deaths could have been prevented by merely providing these children with a few dollars a day of proper food and food supplements. It is also tragic that many malnourished elders die of common infections whereas they probably could have avoided the infection or made a full recovery had they been well nourished.

LUKE CURTIS, MD

Since many nutrients that play a key role in immunity are often deficient in elderly patients, a well-balanced diet with broad-based supplements are needed to produce proper immune function in elders. Several studies of elders in developed nations have reported that supplementation with just one or two nutrients—such as vitamins A, C, and D—are associated with modest 8 to 20% decreases in infection rates as compared to elders who did not receive supplements (Liu 2007; Avenell 2007). Had these patients been supplemented with a broad range of nutrients including many vitamins, minerals, and omega-3, the declines in infection rates would probably have been larger. One study reported that higher consumption of fish and omega-3 fatty acids was associated with significantly lower risk of pneumonia in men aged 44 to 79 years (Merchant 2005).

Cranberries and Cranberry Juice Prevent and Treat Urinary Tract Infections

Urinary tract infections (UTIs) are very common, with about 1 in 4 persons over age 65 years getting at least one UTI per year (Foxman 2002). UTIs are about twice as common in women than men. Many studies have reported that cranberries or cranberry juice can significantly reduce risk of urinary tract infections. Cranberries contain a wide range of phytochemicals called anthocyanins and proanthocyanids, which inhibit growth of bacteria. In four published studies, consumption of cranberries or cranberry juice reduces risk of urinary tract infections by an average of 35% (Jepson 2007). A recent Scottish study of 173 older women with a history of urinary tract infections reported that consumption of cranberry juice extract was as effective as the antibiotic trimethoprim for preventing further UTIs. Moreover, the cranberry juice extract was cheaper and had far fewer adverse side effects than the trimethoprim (McMurdo 2009). Some preliminary evidence suggests that some oral *Lactobacillus* bacteria supplements are useful in reducing the rate of urinary tract infections (Reid 2006). The author urges all elders with recurrent urinary tract infections to consume cranberries or cranberry juice and yogurt or probiotic bacteria regularly.

Milk, yogurt, cheese, and whey protein all contain an excellent assortment of all of the essential amino acids along with antibodies. A number of human and animal studies have associated higher consumption of milk products with stronger immune systems and fewer infections (Yalcin 2006; Weiner 1999). (Whey protein comes from the liquid part of milk after the curds have been separated out to make cheese. Whey protein has a better assortment of amino acids than does the curd protein).

Brazil nuts are an excellent source of the amino acid methionine and the mineral selenium. Both methionine and selenium play a key role in maintaining the body's immune system and in detoxification of harmful chemicals (Thomson 2008). Both methionine and selenium are often low in seniors' diets.

Use of oral probiotic bacteria may also reduce the risk of infections in general. Some, but not all, studies have reported that use of oral probiotic *Lactobacillus* or *Bifidobacterium* reduced incidence of respiratory infections like pneumonia (Vouloumanou 2009). *Lactobacillus* bacteria are commonly found in yogurt. Numerous studies have shown that probiotic bacteria like *Lactobacillus* or *Saccharomyces* can reduce risk of chronic hospital-acquired intestinal infections like *Closteridium difficile*. Please see chapter 7 for more information on probiotics and treatment of hospital-acquired intestinal infections.

Eating a wide variety of fruits and vegetables may also help protect against some infections that grow in the digestive tract. The phytochemicals contained in many fruits and vegetables kill or inhibit growth of many harmful bacteria and yeasts in the intestines (Simoes 2009). For example, vegetables from the Cruciferous family (such as broccoli, cabbage, brussels sprouts) produce phytochemicals such as sulforaphane, which inhibits growth of *Helicobacter* (the bacteria that causes most stomach and intestinal ulcers) and *Candida* in the digestive tract (Johansson 2008). Garlic and onions contain potent phytochemicals such as allicin, which inhibit growth of many harmful bacteria including MRSA (methicillin-resistant *Staphylococcus aureus*) (Fujisawa 2009). In the future, phytochemicals from fruits and vegetables will probably be used much more extensively to fight off common infections.

Nutritional Suggestions to Prevent and/or Reduce Severity of Colds and Flu

Colds are very common viral infections, especially in younger people, but they can also bother the old. About 1 billion cold infections occur annually in the USA (NIAID 2001). Elders average about one cold per year, while young adults average about 2 to 3 per year and children average from 4 to 12 per year (NIAID 2001).

What can be done nutritionally to reduce the risk of colds and flu, or at least reduce the severity of colds and flu? Getting a well-balanced diet with sufficient amounts of water; protein; calories; vitamins (especially A, C, D, and E); minerals (especially zinc); and omega-3 fats are critical for maintaining immunity. Various supplements have been used to try to prevent cold and flu with mixed success. Vitamin C was highly recommended to fight colds by Nobel laureate Linus Pauling in the 1970s. A meta-analysis of thirty studies involving 11,000 subjects reported that supplemental vitamin C had little effect on cold incidence. However, vitamin C supplementation significantly reduced the severity of cold symptoms and significantly reduced the duration of colds by an average of 23% (Douglas, 2007). To improve immunity, most experts recommend taking at least 1,000 milligrams (1 gram) a day of supplemental vitamin C.

Zinc supplements or zinc throat lozenges have often been recommended to fight off colds. A review of eight published studies found mixed results, with four studies reported zinc supplements significantly reduced cold incidence, while four studies found that zinc did not reduce cold incidence (Jackson 2000). A meta-analysis of fourteen studies reported that use of *Echinacea* significantly reduced incidence of colds by an average of 58% (Shah 2007). (*Echinacea* is also known as coneflower and is a common wild and cultivated plant in the US plains). Other supplements, which have had some success in reducing the incidence and/or severity of colds and flu, include N-acetylcysteine (an amino acid), whey protein (from milk), ginseng (Panax), elderberry (*Sambucus nigra*), olive leaf extract, and astragalus (Roxas 2007).

Supplements may not only help prevent infections but also reduce the intensity and length of infections. Broad-based vitamin and mineral supplements are often recommended to elders to help prevent infections. A review of four published studies reported that taking a broad-based multivitamin/mineral supplement had little effect on the rate of all infections in adults older than 65 years (Stephen 2006). However, this same analysis also reported that taking a multivitamin/mineral supplement was associated with an average of sixteen fewer days of infection as compared to those not taking the supplement (results very statistically significant). Antibiotic use was also significantly reduced in the elders taking the broad-based multivitamin and mineral supplement (Stephen 2006).

Handwashing Can Prevent Colds and Flu

Handwashing is also a critical step in preventing spread of cold and flu. Be sure to wash hands in soap and water for at least fifteen seconds after coughing, sneezing, handshaking, and before activities such as eating or putting your hands to

LUKE CURTIS, MD

your face. Use of alcohol-based hand cleaners are also effective against cold and flu viruses. Several school studies have reported that programs to encourage handwashing significantly reduce absenteeism due to colds and flu among both elementary students and college students (White 2005; Guinan 2002).

Many types of hand soaps and alcohol-based hand disinfecting products are available. The author encourages seniors to try several varieties and pick the brand they like best. The chemicals in some soaps and alcohol-based disinfectants may irritate some people's skin and may also trigger asthmatic symptoms in some people if heavily scented.

Nutrition to Combat Myelodysplasia: A Form of Bone Marrow Failure that Can Greatly Increase Infection Risk

A fairly common problem that can cause reduced immunity to infection in elders is myelodysplasia or bone marrow failure. Myelodysplasia occurs in about 1 in 2,000 people over the age of 70 years (Aul 1998). Myelodysplasia involves failure of the bone marrow to manufacture red blood cells, white blood cells, and platelets. The bone marrow that makes red blood cells are responsible for transporting oxygen from the lungs to the cells and for transporting carbon dioxide from the cells to be exhaled by the lungs. The bone marrow also makes white blood cells, which fight infections and platelets that help blood to clot. People with myelodysplasia suffer fatigue, weakened resistance to infection, problems with blood clotting, and poorer wound healing.

Some myelodysplasia involve leukemia and other types of cancer. Anyone with myelodysplasia should get a thorough medical workup to rule out cancer. However, many cases of myelodysplasia are nutritional in nature and respond well to a better diet and supplements. Myelodysplasia can be caused by deficiencies of many nutrients including protein, calories, zinc, iron, copper, vitamin B_{12}, folate (a B vitamin), vitamins C and E, and L-carnitine (an amino acid) (Curtis 2008b). Copper deficiency is especially common in patients on tube-feeding (enteral) formulas (Curtis 2008b).

Patients with nutritionally related myelodysplasia should receive a well-balanced diet with ample amounts of water, protein, calories, omega-3 fats, and fruits/vegetables. Myelodysplasia patients should also receive a good daily multivitamin mineral supplement that contains at least 15 milligrams of zinc, 10 milligrams of iron, and 2 milligrams of copper. However, iron should be given with caution in patients who have received many blood transfusions, as many blood transfusions can cause iron overload. The daily supplements should also contain at least 50 micrograms of vitamin B_{12}, 400 milligrams of folate, 500 milligrams of vitamin C, 400 international units (IU) of vitamin E, and at least 1,000 milligrams of L-carnitine (Curtis 2008b). For more information and suggestions for supplements, please see chapter 18. The author has seen several patients in their eighties and nineties with noncancer-related myelodysplasia improve dramatically when given a good diet and a good multivitamin mineral supplement containing copper, zinc, and iron. These patients not only showed increases in their red blood cell, white blood cell, and platelet counts but also had a huge increase in energy and had fewer illnesses.

The next chapter will focus on nutrition for hospitalized patients.

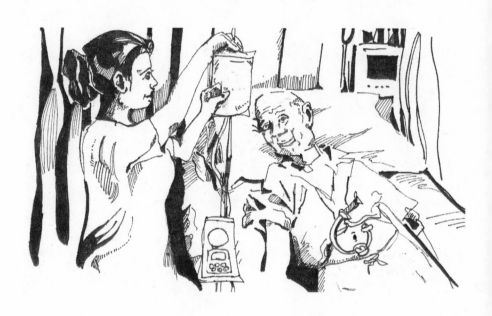

CHAPTER 7

BETTER HOSPITAL NUTRITION
IS CRITICAL FOR RECOVERY

Most Hospitalized Elders Are Badly Malnourished

Hospital nutrition is important to promote healing from persons recovering from surgery, cancer, heart disease, accidents, and other serious health problems. However, the majority of hospitalized elderly are badly malnourished. As noted earlier, five large published studies have reported that from 42 to 91% of hospitalized patients over age 65 years are badly malnourished and lacking in protein and calories (Kubrak and Jensen 2007). A large study of 630 hospitalized patients reported that hospital-acquired infections were five times as common in malnourished versus well-nourished patients (Schneider 2004).

Besides having protein-calories malnutrition, most elderly hospitalized patients are also low in many nutrients including omega-3 fats and many vitamins and minerals (Wintergerst 2007). The high rates of malnutrition in hospitalized patients and the higher rates of infections and other complications in hospitalized patients who were malnourished was recognized as long ago as 1859 by the famous nurse Florence Nightingale (Nightingale 1859).

Hospital nutrition is critical for recovery for many infections, illnesses, and injuries. Proper nutrition can often mean the difference between death and good recovery for many elderly patients. However, as noted in chapter 2, most physicians have very little education or interest in nutritional issues (Adams 2004). Malnutrition is found in at least 42% of all elder hospitalized patents, yet this malnutrition is documented in medical charts for less than 1 in 1,100 malnourished patients (Bobcock 2009).

Family and friends can often help the hospitalized senior to eat and give them food supplements. For patients who cannot eat food by mouth, prompt tube feeding can greatly reduce infection, death, and other complications. Family members of patients unable to eat by regular routes can urge physicians and nurses to promptly give the patient a high-quality tube (enteral) "immunonutrition" feeding formula.

The previous chapter on nutrition and infection noted that malnutrition greatly reduces immunity and increases chance of infection. This chapter will discuss nutritional and non-nutritional methods of greatly reducing hospital-acquired infections. Poor hospital nutrition is responsible for many of the 100,000 annual US deaths due to hospital-acquired infection (Curtis 2008). Poor hospital nutrition is also responsible for poorer wound healing and poorer function of the heart, lungs, kidneys, and other organs (Kubrak and Jensen 2007).

Good Diet, Supplements, and Nutritional Drinks Helpful for Hospitalized Patients

Many jokes exist about hospital food. The author remembers all sorts of jokes in medical school about the quality of hospital food. "This greeting card was made of recycled hospital

LUKE CURTIS, MD

jello" reads one popular get-well card. However, the effects of malnutrition on increasing hospital complications are no joke at all.

Hospitalized patients who are able to eat regular food should be encouraged to eat at least three well-balanced meals daily. Each meal should contain a high-quality protein source like meat, fish, eggs, or milk/yogurt. At least eight cups of fluids (water, milk, smoothies, coffee, tea, etc.) should be obtained, unless the patient is on a water-restricted diet. Patients should eat at least five servings of fruits and vegetables if tolerated.

Many institutions are making a good effort to improve the quality of hospital food. If hospitalized elders have favorite foods, it is often possible for the hospital kitchen to prepare them if given advanced notice. Family members can also provide favorite high-nutrition foods like nuts and cheese to the patients.

Supplements are also important for hospitalized elderly. In general, patients should consume the same supplements they were consuming at home. Yogurt or capsules of probiotic bacteria are especially useful for those who had multiple courses of antibiotics (please see chapter 13 for more information on probiotics). Supplements of vitamins A, C,D, B complex, zinc, copper, and selenium are especially helpful for patients battling infections (please see chapter 6, "Nutrition to Prevent and Treat Infection"). Amino acid supplements of glutamine, arginine, and leucine are often especially useful for burn/trauma/surgical patients or patients with extensive muscle loss (please see chapter 4, "Nutrition and Exercise for Treating Muscle Loss (Sarcopenia)").

Providing feeding assistance can often be very helpful to hospitalized patients who are not eating. In medical school, the author remembered seeing a 91-year old woman from Puerto Rico who was getting weaker every day and had lost 40 pounds in four months. She was eating little of the food on her hospital tray. However, she was able to eat two entire lunches in a row with his help. Helping her was somewhat of a challenge since she spoke only Spanish and his knowledge of Spanish is limited. He then instructed her daughter and grandchildren to help her eat meals at home. Two months later, the patient had gained back 20 pounds and was feeling much stronger.

Another way to improve nutritional intake for seniors with a poor appetite in hospital or at home is the use of nutritional drinks like Boost (Nestlé Company) or Ensure (Abbott Labs). These drinks are available in many flavors and contain balanced amounts of water, protein, fats, carbohydrates, vitamins, minerals, and fiber. Some of the newer drinks like Peptamen (Nestlé) contain additional important ingredients such as glutamine or omega-3 fatty acids. Some of these nutritional drinks contain a fair amount of sugar and may not be appropriate for diabetics. Special low-sugar drinks like Glucerna (Nestlé) are available for diabetic persons. A number of studies have reported that use of such nutritional drinks among elders in hospitals/care centers is associated with a higher intake of protein, calories, vitamins, and minerals and are also associated with significantly faster wound healing and significant lower rates of infection and death (Johnson 2009).

Such drinks are available in a number of flavors such as chocolate, vanilla, strawberry, and banana. The author remembers caring for a thin 78-year-old hospitalized man with advanced lung cancer. He had some difficulties in eating and was given vanilla Boost. He said he preferred the chocolate flavor but the hospital had only vanilla. The author bought him a six-pack of chocolate Boost, and later his family bought him chocolate Boost. The man drank far more of the chocolate Boost than vanilla Boost and gained a few pounds. Such nutritional drinks like Boost or Ensure are often useful for elderly folks at home. They make a good replacement for colas, coffee, and tea for malnourished elders.

LUKE CURTIS, MD

Burn, Trauma, and Major Surgery Patients Need Special Nutritional Support

Patients who have undergone major burns, major trauma from an accident, or major surgery need specialized nutrition. Nutritional needs for water, protein, calories, omega-3 and omega-6 fats, and many vitamins and minerals are greatly increased in these patients (Gudaviciene 2004). Levels of minerals like zinc, copper, and selenium are often very low in burn patients. A numbers of studies have reported that supplementing burn patients diets with four to six times the usual levels of zinc, copper, and selenium is helping in speeding healing times (Gudaviciene 2004). Burn patients are also often low in vitamins A, C, D, and B complex and can benefit from supplementation (Gudaviciene 2004). Consuming cod-liver oil in burn patients has also been associated with shorter healing times and significantly fewer infections (Gudaviciene 2004). Supplementation with the amino acids glutamine and arginine can also be very helpful in burn patients (Andel 2003).

Levels of fluids and insulin also needs to be carefully monitored in burn patients. Any patient with burns over 20% of their body and/or severe traumatic injuries should receive specialized nutritional care and counseling within twenty-four hours of the burn injury.

Everyone should be concerned about preventing fires and fire injuries. Every year, about 900 people in the USA over age 65 years die of fires and smoke exposure (CDC 2006). About 25% of fatal fires are caused by smoking accidents (Fire Safety 2010). All smokers should consider joining a smoking cessation group. If smokers are unwilling to quit, they should at least limit their smoking to outdoors to reduce indoor fire and health risks.

All homes, apartments, and senior centers should have fire extinguishers and smoke alarms. Batteries in smoke alarms should be check regularly and replaced if low. Seniors need to pay special attention to avoid cooking fires. Use of electric stoves has a lower risk of fires than gas stoves.

In the author's opinion, use of candles, fireplaces, wood-burning stoves, and burning of leaves/grass/trash are a major fire risk and should be avoided. Wood-burning stoves and fireplaces are both fire risks and severely pollute the air (Curtis 2002). Burning of leaves and brush also presents a serious fire danger to people of all ages, and these materials should be composted instead (Wibbenmeyer 2003). The author has seen several formerly healthy elderly people badly burned from cigarette, candle, or leaf-burning fires.

Prompt Tube Feeding (Enteral Nutrition) Is Oftentimes Critical in Hospital Recovery and Avoiding Complications and Death

Many people in the hospital cannot eat food by the regular route by mouth and must be given tube feeding (enteral feeding) via a tube in their nasal passages or by a small hole made in the stomach or intestine. A common procedure to feed patients who cannot eat by the normal route is called a percutaneous endoscopic gastronomy or simply PEG. A PEG tube can be made to make a feeding line in the stomach in minor surgical procedure that takes about ten minutes and does not require general anesthesia. PEG insertion is a low-risk procedure, which usually can be performed even in very ill patients (Zippi 2009).

Much research has indicated that early and proper tube-feeding nutrition can reduce risk of infection and death among hospitalized patients and enable most to return to eating regularly by mouth. Tube feeding must begin soon after an ill patient stops eating. Delaying feeding for three to ten days is very commonly done and can greatly increase risk of infection and death for the patient (Kubrak and Jensen 2007). Such three

LUKE CURTIS, MD

to ten days delays in feeding can greatly deplete levels of many of the body's nutrients and greatly lower immunity and greatly increase risk of infection (Wintergerst 2007). In other words, even a few days without nutrition can greatly reduce the ability of the body to fight infection.

Benefits of tube-feeding patients can quickly greatly reduce risk of death, infection, and other complications. For example, a recent meta-analysis of six published studies has reported that tube-feeding patients within twenty-four hours of injury or intensive care unit (ICU) reduces risk of death by 66% as compared to patients whose tube feeding was delayed! (Doig 2009). Incidence of pneumonia was reduced 69% in patients receiving tube feeding within twenty-four hours as compared to patients whose tube feeding was delayed. Incidence of multiple organ failure syndrome was reduced by 60% in patients given the early tube feeding. (Multiple organ failure syndrome involved failure of several organs such as heart, liver, kidneys, and brain). All of these lower levels of death and complications seen in these studies were very statistically significant (Doig 2009).

Surgery patients are often kept without any oral or tube feeding for three to ten days (Mattei 2006). Many physicians and surgeons insist upon not feeding any patient who does not have bowel sounds and producing gas. However, recent studies have suggested that even in patients with no bowel sounds, virtually all patients can be given either regular food or tube feeding within forty-eight hours of surgery. The main exceptions are those with major stomach or intestinal surgery who might need some time to rebuilding their gut. (These patients can be fed intravenously until their gut rebuilds.) Several studies report that "fast-track" enteral feeding of surgical patients with forty-eight hours of surgery speeds recovery and significantly reduces risk of infection and death (Mattei 2006).

In medical school, the author was often frustrated to see many surgical and intensive care patients get weaker and get many infections when kept without nutrition unnecessarily for three to ten days. On the other hand, he saw many patients who were given tube feeding immediately. Most of these patients who received prompt tube feeding got better quickly, started walking with a week, resumed normal eating, and left the hospital within two weeks.

Enriched "Immunonutrition" Tube Feeding Formulas Significantly Reduce Risk of Infection

While early feeding with tube formulas can speed recovery, reduce risk of infection and death, better quality formulas such as "immunonutrition" formulas, which can also speed recovery and reduce risk of complications. In recent years, immunonutrition enteral formulas have been developed, which contain larger quantities of antioxidant vitamins, zinc and other minerals, omega-3 fatty acids, and amino acids like glutamine. Brand names of these immunonutrition formulas include Peptamen AF, Impact, Crucial (all three from Nestlé/Novartis), Oxepa and Optimental (Abbott), and Stressen (Nutricia) (Marik 2008).

Meta-analysis has calculated that tube-fed (enteral) immunonutrition in hospitalized patients is associated with a 46% lower risk of hospital-acquired pneumonia (eleven studies), a 55% lower risk of acute bacterial infection (nine studies), a 78% lower risk of abdominal abscess infections (six studies), and a 34% lower risk of urinary tract infections (ten studies) compared with patients receiving standard tube (enteral) formulas (Montejo et al. 2003). All of these analyses of studies gave statistically very significant results.

Use of immunonutrition tube formulas can be very helpful in correcting the severe nutritional deficiencies seen in most hospitalized elderly. A recent study of ICU patients with severe infections provided twenty-seven with an "immunonutrition" formula (containing extra amounts of zinc, selenium, vitamins C

LUKE CURTIS, MD

and E, beta-carotene, the amino acids glutamine and arginine, and omega-3 fatty acids) and gave twenty-eight patients standard formula (Beale 2008). At the start of study, average blood levels of many nutrients such as vitamins C, E, beta-carotene, zinc, and selenium were abnormally low. After ten days of treatment, multiple organ function (heart, lungs, liver, kidney) was significantly better in the immunonutrition group as compared to the standard nutrition group, and blood levels of many nutrients improved at a significantly faster rate in the immunonutrition group. Infection rates were also significantly lower in the patients who received the extra nutrition via the immunonutrition formula (Beale 2008).

Probiotic Bacteria and Yeasts Fight Infections in Tube Fed Patients

Many hospitalized patients develop serious infections in the intestines by a bad bacteria called *Closteridium difficile* after several antibiotic courses. *Closteridium difficile* can frequently cause life-threatening infections. Probiotic bacteria and yeasts can be helpful in preventing or clearing infections by *Closteridium difficile* and other bacteria. Such probiotic organisms can be given by mouth or in tube feeds. Probiotic bacteria used include *Lactobacillus* and *Bifidobacterium*, which are found in yogurt while probiotic yeasts include *Saccharomyces*, which is used to raise bread.

Meta-analysis of twenty-five studies reported that supplemental *Saccharomyces boulardii*, *Lactobacillus* spp., or *Bifidobacterium* spp. were associated with significantly lower levels of antibiotic-associated diarrhea (McFarland 2006). Meta-analysis of six studies indicated that *S. boulardii* was effective in reducing the incidence of *Closteridium difficile* diarrhea (McFarland 2006). Yogurt containing active *Lactobacillus* spp. has been found to be effective in preventing or clearing infections caused by

Closteridium difficile and VRE in hospitalized patients (Hickson 2007; Manley 2007).

Probiotic bacteria are frequently included in tube feeds to patients being given enteral (tube) nutrition (DeLegge 2008). Probiotic bacteria are available in hospital pharmacies or over-the-counter without a prescription in health food stores. More information about probiotic or good bacteria will be given in chapter 13 on digestive health in elderly.

Family Members Should Urge Immunonutrition Formulas and Probiotics for Their Tube-Fed Relatives

Family members should instruct the medical staff to give the tube-fed hospitalized senior the highly nutritious "immunonutrition" formulas and also consider giving probiotic or "good" bacteria (such as *Lactobacillus* and *Bifidobacterium*) to reduce risk of intestinal infections. As noted above, such immunonutrition formulas include Peptamen AF, Impact, Crucial (all three from Nestlé/Novartis), Oxepa and Optimental (Abbott), and Stressen (Nutricia) (Marik 2008). Some of these Formulas (Peptamen and Optimental) also contain partially digested whey (milk) proteins and partially digested fats (short chain fatty acids), which are easier for critically ill patients to digest. Feeding such immunonutrition formulas can often mean the difference between good recovery and death to many critically ill patients.

Tube-fed hospitalized patients with special needs like diabetes or fluid restrictions may need modifications of some of these nutritional formulas. If patient can't receive an immunonutrition formula for some reason, they should at least receive a vitamin/mineral supplement and at least 1 teaspoon a day or fish or cod-liver oil via tube. Fish oil is commonly given, added to feeding tube formulas and/or given directly in the feeding tube. A review of fifteen published studies reported that supplementation with fish oil significantly reduced death rates by 58% in hospitalized tube fed patients! (Marik 2008).

The use of better tube-feeding formulas can have dramatic effects on improving very ill patients. The author was involved with a man who was a ballet dancer in his twenties, was later a math professor for 42 years, and was very healthy until age 88. At 88, he entered the hospital for minor surgery and developed nine (!) hospital-acquired infections. He was placed on a ventilator, tube feeding, and kidney dialysis. The physicians advised "pulling the plug" and letting the patient die. The author saw the patient was badly malnourished and sarcopenic. He suggested improving his tube feeding by switching to Pepteman AF formula with fish oil and start physical/speech therapy. This Peptamen HP formula contained partially digested whey protein, partially digested coconut oil, fish oil, and higher levels of vitamins and minerals than most tube-feeding (enteral) formulas. Following better nutrition, physical therapy, exercise, and lots of encouragement to the patient, the 88-year-old patient was able to discontinue the ventilator, kidney dialysis, and tube feeding; resume normal eating; and return home. A year later, the patient was walking one mile a day! The patient was well enough to write and publish an article in the *Dancing Times* (London) about the great dancer/ choreographer Leonide Massine during his convalescence!

Handwashing and Non-Nutritional Methods to Reduce the 100,000 US Annual Deaths Due to Hospital-Acquired Infections

Besides nutrition, what can patients or their families do to reduce the risk of hospital-acquired infection? Patients and family members should insist that all physicians, nurses, and staff who visit wash their hands with soap or water or alcohol-based solution. Many published studies have reported that less half of physicians and nurses wash their hands before seeing patients! Many studies have reported that programs to increase handwashing among physicians and nurses have significantly lower hospital-acquired infections rates (Curtis 2008). Wearing gloves, gowns, and shoe covers can also reduce risk of hospital-acquired infection rates.

When patients have to undergo surgery, choosing the least invasive surgery can reduce risk of infection. For example, many surgeries can be done laparoscopically instead of making a huge open incision in the patient. Laparoscopic surgery involves making three small holes in the patient and visualizing the internal organs with fiber optics. Many studies have reported that laparoscopic surgery has much lower rates of infection than open surgeries (Curtis 2008). Most abdominal surgeries, some lung and heart surgeries, and even knee replacement surgeries can now be done laparoscopically.

Air filters in rooms can significantly reduce risk of airborne hospital infections. Use of urinary and blood catheters containing antiseptic silver compounds can significantly reduce risk of hospital-acquired infections (Curtis 2008). Catheters are plastic tubes used in hospitals to drain urine and give fluids and blood to patients.

The author has published on a sixteen-page review forty-eight methods to reduce hospital-acquired infections in the July 2008 *Journal of Hospital Infection*. Readers wishing to obtain a free copy of this paper are welcome to contact me at LukeTCurtis@ aol.com.

The next two chapters will concentrate on using nutrition to prevent and treat the most common life-threatening illnesses in elders including heart disease, strokes and lung problems (chapter 8), and cancer (chapter 9).

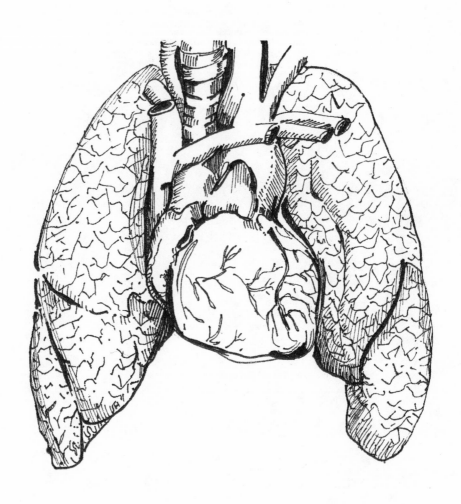

CHAPTER 8

NUTRITION TO IMPROVE HEART, CARDIOVASCULAR, AND LUNG HEALTH AND PREVENT HEART DISEASE, STROKE, AND ASTHMA

The condition of the heart, blood vessels, and lungs are critical for maintaining optimal health. Every day, your heart beats about 100,000 times and pushes about 7,500 quarts (7,000 liters) of blood through about 100,000 miles of blood vessels and capillaries (capillaries are tiny blood vessels just large enough for one red or white blood cell to pass) (Berne 1998). Every day, your lungs breathe about 28,000 times and process about 700 cubic feet (20 cubic meters) of air (Berne 1998).

Proper nutrition, sufficient exercise, and avoidance of smoking can do wonders to keep these organs functioning well and avoiding heart disease, stroke, and lung problems. Problems with the heart, vascular system, and lungs cause a lot of death and disability in the USA. Annually in the United States, heart disease causes about 631,000 deaths, strokes about 137,000, and respiratory failure about 124,000 deaths (Heron 2009).

Quitting Smoking at Any Age Greatly Reduces Risk of Heart Disease, Strokes, and Breathing Problems Like Asthma and Emphysema

Ten percent of US adults over age 65 years were smoking in 2007 (Doolan 2008). Smoking is a major risk factor for heart disease, strokes, kidney disease, atherosclerosis (hardening of the arteries), dementia, and respiratory problems like asthma and emphysema. Studies report that quitting smoking even in sixties or seventies can have major health benefits including reduced risk of heart disease, lung cancer, and emphysema and significantly longer life expectancy (Taylor 2002). Much research has found that using nicotine patches/gum and/or stop-smoking groups are helpful for older adults who want to quit (Andrews 2000). Older smokers have the best success rate of quitting smoking of any age group. Over 70% of smokers older than 65 years who try to quit smoking are successful, even though it may take several tries to quit successfully (Doolan 2008). Most persons who quit smoking take several tries, so do not lose heart if you backslide into smoking once or twice or thrice briefly.

The author strongly urges all smokers to investigate stop-smoking groups in their communities. Many hospitals, public health clinics, businesses, and religious groups offer stop-smoking groups and seminars. A listing on online stop-smoking groups is available at http://www.google.com/Top/Health/Support_Groups/Smoking_Cessation/.

Even exposure to secondhand tobacco smoke is bad for cardiovascular and lung health. A meta-analysis of ten studies in four nations reported that heart attack rates were 30% higher in nonsmoker married to smokers versus nonsmokers (Glantz 1990). Many studies have reported that exposure to secondhand smoke can worsen and/or increase risk of asthma, bronchitis, emphysema, lung infections, and stroke in elderly patients (Jaakkola 2002).

LUKE CURTIS, MD

Other Environmental Exposures
May Trigger Health Problems

Hundreds of published studies have reported that exposure to low to moderate levels of many outdoor air pollutants such as particulates (PM), ozone, and carbon monoxide can significantly increase rates of heart disease, strokes, hardening of the arteries (atherosclerosis), and asthma (Curtis 2006). Dozens of studies have reported that exposure to molds and pollen can also worsen rates of asthma and nasal problems (Curtis 2004). Perfumes, pesticides, formaldehyde, and many other indoor air pollutants have also been linked to worsen asthma (Shim 1986).

Nutrition to Prevent and Treat Heart Attacks
and Heart Failure

Heart disease is very common in elders, with about 29% of US adults over age 80 years having some form of heart disease (American Heart Association 2009). While heart disease is usually thought of as man's disease, after menopause, women die of heart disease at a rate similar to that of men (American Heart Association 2009).

Diet plays a key role in preventing heart disease. The following dietary interventions have been found to significantly reduce risk of heart disease: lower saturated fat reduced heart disease risk in two of nine studies, lower trans-fat acids in four of four studies, higher omega-3 fats in three of three studies, higher fiber consumption in four of four studies, higher nut consumption in five of six studies, higher fruits and vegetables in seven of eight studies, and high level of whole grains in four of four studies (Hu 2002). Several studies have reported that high consumption of citrus fruits (oranges, grapefruits) can reduce risk of heart disease and improve health of blood vessels (Benavente-Garcia 2008).

Meta-analysis of nine studies reported that consumption of 700 milligrams or more supplemental vitamin C daily was associated with lower rates of coronary heart disease, while higher vitamin E and beta-carotene consumption was associated with marginally lower rates of coronary heart disease (Knekt 2004). Another analysis of fifteen studies reported that consuming supplements containing 30 international units of more of vitamin E significantly reduced risk of heart attacks (Ye 2008). On the other hand, another review reported that use of antioxidant supplements was associated with a significantly improved cardiovascular outcome in five studies, no significant difference in outcome in ten studies, and significantly worse outcome in five studies (Kris-Etherton 2004). A review of six studies reported that daily supplementation with 75 or 100 micrograms of selenium daily was associated with a 11% lower risk of heart attacks (Flores-Mateo 2006).

Nutrition plays a vital role in helping people who have already have heart problems. Several studies have reported that among recent heart attack patients, oral or intravenous supplements of magnesium were associated with significantly lower death rates (Shechter 2005). Two studies have reported that consumption of omega-3 fatty acids in patients with preexisting heart disease is associated with significantly fewer coronary events and significantly lower coronary or all cause mortality (Burr 1989; Marchioli 2001). Several studies have also reported that supplemental omega-3 fats are associated with significantly lower rates of heartbeat irregularities (Lavie 2009). Other studies showed that a low-fat diet did not significantly reduce coronary events in patients with previous heart attacks (myocardial infarctions) (Burr 1989; Ball 1985). Higher nut consumption has been associated with significantly fewer coronary events for patients with previous heart attacks (Brown 1999).

Heart failure is a common condition in which the heart becomes less efficient in pumping blood to the body. Heart failure is treated with a number of drugs such as water pills (diuretics) or drugs that lower blood pressure such as ACE inhibitors (such as Capoten, Vasotec, Zestril, Univasc, and Altace). Generally drug treatment is only moderately successful for heart failure.

Many heart failure patients are low in many nutrients including potassium, calcium, magnesium, zinc, B vitamins, coenzyme Q_{10}, and amino acids such as L-carnitine, creatine, and L-taurine. Many of these nutrients are needed for optimum functioning of the muscle cells in the heart. A number of studies have reported that broad-based supplementation with a wide range of nutrients including magnesium, zinc, high dose B complex vitamins, and coenzyme Q_{10} can often help improve heart function in heart failure patients. Such a supplementation regime can improve the metabolic pathways in the heart muscle cells, thereby improving pumping efficiency of the heart and reducing the problems associated with heart failure (Soukoulis 2009).

Heart failure diets need a well-balanced diet with a good source of protein three times daily (lean meat, fish, poultry, low-fat dairy products) and at least five servings a day of a wide variety of fruits and vegetables. The high level of potassium found in fruits and vegetables improve heart function and control high blood pressure. Heart failure patients should also get a good nutritional supplementation program, which includes ample zinc, magnesium, potassium, B vitamins, coenzyme Q_{10}, and amino acids such as taurine, creatine, and L-carnitine. One supplement that has been used successfully in several published studies to significantly improve heart function in heart failure patients is called MyoVive. A one day's dose of this broad-based formula contains 3.0 grams of L-carnitine, 150 milligrams of coenzyme Q_{10}, 3.0 grams of taurine, 2.25 grams of creatine, 750 milligrams of potassium, 15 milligrams of zinc, and fairly high doses of B vitamins including 25 milligrams of thiamine (B_1) (Jeejeebhoy 2002).

Dramatic improvements in heart health can often occur in older adults who improve their diet, stop smoking, and get more exercise. The author had one patient who suffered a severe heart attack at age 68 years and required five-way (quintuple) heart bypass surgery. Following the heart attack and bypass, he quit smoking "cold turkey" and ate a well-balanced diet emphasizing fruits and vegetables, fish, lean meats, low-fat dairy products, and whole grains. He also began taking food supplements including a good multivitamin mineral supplement and 1 tablespoon of cod-liver oil, 400 milligrams of magnesium, 75 milligrams of zinc, 100 milligrams of coenzyme Q_{10}, and 2,000 milligrams of L-carnitine daily. He then gradually increased his exercise and now is riding his bicycle 100 to 300 miles per week and lifting weights three times a week. At 72, he is now working full-time in a business position. He now has more energy than many men half his age. This patient is now trying to convince his 42-year-old son to stop smoking, improve his diet, and begin exercising. The author knows many children who improved their diet, stopped smoking, and begin exercising after seeing what a huge health improvement that these lifestyle interventions had made in their parents.

Exercise, Social and Religious Support, Sex, and Pets Are Helpful for Maintaining Heart Health

Even small amounts of exercise can greatly increase heart and lung capacity in middle-aged and older folks. A French study had nineteen formerly sedentary older adults (average age 65 years) work out on a stationary bike for thirty minutes for twice a week. After nine weeks of workouts, the average heart and lung capacity increased by an average of 10%! (Lepretre 2009). An increase in heart and lung capacity of 10% means that a 65-year-old person has heart and lungs about as strong as a sedentary person ten or twenty years younger! *It is amazing that exercising only one hour per week can make an older person's heart and lungs ten to twenty years younger in capacity!*

Many communities have medically supervised heart (cardiac) rehabilitation programs.

Many studies have reported that these heart rehabilitation programs can significantly reduce risk of dying from a second heart attack and can also significantly improve blood pressure and cholesterol levels and significantly reduce the depression commonly seen in patients recovering from a heart attack (Taylor 2004; Eshah,2009). Such programs provide much social support and encouragement. The author encourages all heart patients to consider joining a cardiovascular rehabilitation program.

Social support from spouses, friends, relatives, and social and religious organizations are also important for preventing and treating heart problems. Many studies have reported that people with a low level of social support have about a 50% to 100% increased risk of getting an initial or second heart attack (Lett 2005). Another study reported that belonging to a religious group was associated with significantly better health and significantly lower death rate in elderly who had undergone heart operations (Oxman 1995). Lonely elders should consider joining a social, religious, or exercise group for more social contacts. Walking, bicycle, exercise class, and dance classes are especially helpful since they provide both needed social support and exercise. Single elderly people should consider joining dating clubs or a dating service. Dating services now abound to help middle-aged and elderly folks find sweethearts. For example the dating site Match.com has 2.5 million members over the age of 55 (webpersonals.online 2009).

Sexual intimacy is generally very safe and pleasant for heart patients and can significantly reduce risk for heart attacks. A recent study of 1,165 middle-aged and older men reported that those who had sexual activity at least twice a week had a 45% lower risk of heart disease as compared to men with sex less than once a month (Hall 2010). Results were adjusted for such factors as age and health status.

Erectile dysfunction or impotence is common in older men, with about 35% of men over age 70 years having erectile dysfunction all or most of the time (Selvin 2007). Damage to blood vessels is the most common cause of both heart disease and erectile dysfunction in men. The biggest risk factors for erectile dysfunction in the elderly are smoking and diabetes, and quitting smoking and controlling diabetes can also improve erectile dysfunction (Selvin 2007). The new phosphodiesterase medications such as Viagra, Levitra, and Cialis are very effective in improving erectile function in men from age 65 to 100 years (Sharlip 2008).

Nutrition and supplements can also be useful for treating impotence. One study involved switching thirty-five middle-aged men with severe erectile dysfunction to a Mediterranean Diet rich in fruits, vegetables, fish, whole grains, nuts, and oil olive. The men were not given any specific drugs for erectile dysfunction. After two years on the Mediterranean Diet, thirteen of the men regained full erectile function and most of the remaining twenty-two reported some improvement in erectile function (Esposito 2006). Other studies have reported that daily supplementation with 2 grams a day of carnitine of 6 grams a day of arginine can also significantly improve erectile function in men over 60 year old (Cavallini 2004; Chen 1999).

Nutrition can also help sexual function in postmenopausal women. One study of forty-nine menopausal women with low sexual desire reported that women given a supplement containing multivitamins, minerals, arginine, ginseng, and ginkgo for four weeks had much better sexual function than women given placebo. Symptoms, which improved significantly in the supplement group, included a better sex drive, more frequent sexual intercourse, and less vaginal dryness (Ito 2006). Other studies have reported that testosterone therapy can significantly improve sexual function in postmenopausal women with low testosterone (Hubayter 2008). Some, but not all studies, have

LUKE CURTIS, MD

reported that supplementation soy protein can also improve such menopausal problems as loss of sexual drive, vaginal dryness, depression, and hot flashes (Albert 2002).

Pets can also provide important support for both heart and mental health. A New York study of heart attack survivors found that owning a pet dog was associated with a significantly increased level of survivorship for a year following the heart attack (Friedman 1995). Another study reported that cat ownership was associated with a 30% lower risk of heart attack risk in middle-aged and older adults (Paddock 2008). Many pets, especially dogs, are useful in that they encourage adults to getting more walking exercise. One study noted that dog owners get considerably more walking exercise than non-dog owners (Yabroff 2008).

Pet dogs and cats make especially good companions for elders who are widowed or have a spouse with dementia. Various studies have reported that ownership of dogs and cats can reduce depression and anxiety in elders (Likourezos 2002). Millions of loveable dogs and cats are now waiting in shelters to be adopted. The author urges all elders who are pet lovers to consider adopting a dog and/or cat. On the negative side, dogs and cats require a fair amount of time and money to maintain and may cause severe grief if they die or become seriously ill.

Nutrition and Stroke Prevention

While strokes ("brain attacks") can occur at any age, strokes are far more common in elders. About 15% of US adults over the age of 70 have suffered at least one stroke (American Heart Association 2009). As with heart disease, good nutrition can play a major role in stroke prevention. However, nutritional research on strokes is much sparser than nutritional research for heart disease.

Eating more fruits and vegetables and/or following a Mediterranean Diet are associated with significantly lower rates of stroke (He 2006; Spence 2006). The Mediterranean Diet is rich in fruits, vegetables, fish, whole grains, and olive oil. Some studies have reported that consumption of fish, fish oil, B vitamins, and antioxidant vitamins such as A, C, and E are associated with lower stroke risk, while many studies have reported no association between these nutrients and stroke risk (Spence 2006; Sanchez-Moreno 2009). Why do fruits and vegetables seem to be more effective in preventing stroke than supplements of antioxidant vitamins like A and C? It may be because fruits and vegetables are not only rich in vitamins A and C, but also contain many phytochemicals that have beneficial effects on the circulatory system.

A large Australian study of 665 middle-aged and elderly men reported that consumption of two or more glasses of milk daily was associated with a 48% lower risk of stroke (results statistically significant) (Elwood 2005).

Many studies have reported that treating high blood and high LDL cholesterol lower rates of stroke and reduce risk of a second stroke (American Heart Association 2009). Later in this chapter, the relationships between nutrition, high blood pressure, and high LDL cholesterol levels will be examined in detail.

Following a stroke, many patients may have difficulty eating and may need assistance at meals. Malnutrition is significantly higher in stroke patients who have eating difficulties but get no eating assistance (Foley 2009). Getting swallowing and speech therapy can be very helpful to help stroke patients resume eating normally (Logemann 2007). The author has seen many stroke patients who had trouble eating following a stroke and who required eating assistance or tube feeding (see chapter 7 for tube-feeding information) resume eating normally following a program of good nutrition and swallowing therapy.

LUKE CURTIS, MD

Nutrition to Slow Progression of Hardening and Filling of Arteries

Most people have some hardening of the arteries or atherosclerosis by the time they reach middle age and beyond. Atherosclerosis involves thickening and filling up the arteries with cholesterol, dead cells, and fibers or plaques. (Arteries are blood vessels traveling from the heart, while veins are vessels traveling to the heart.) Severe atherosclerosis can block important arteries and put patients at much greater risk for heart disease, strokes, kidney failure, and dementia (American Heart Association 2010).

The left and right carotid arteries are two of only four arteries that supply blood to the head (the other two are the vertebral arteries). Blockage of these carotid arteries puts patients at much greater risk of stroke. The thickness and degree of atherosclerosis of these arteries can easily be assayed by ultrasound. Patients with over 60% blockage of these arteries are usually advised to use diet and medication to reduce atherosclerosis, while patients with over 75% blockage are usually advised to have surgery to clean out the carotid arteries.

Diet and exercise can play a major role in preventing atherosclerosis buildup in vital arteries such as in the carotid arteries and the coronary (heart) arteries. A number of research studies have examined the effects of diet on carotid artery atherosclerosis in middle-aged and older adults. Consumption of five or more fruits and vegetables daily, eating two or more servings of fish weekly, eating 2 tablespoons of olive oil per day, getting a daily supplement of 610 milligrams of magnesium, and getting regular exercise were all associated with significant lower rates of atherosclerosis or filling up of the carotid arteries (Ellingsen 2009; Erkkila 2004; Buil-Cosiales 2008; Turgut 2008; Wildman 2004). Cigarette smoking is associated with much faster rates of atherosclerosis and artery blockage (Baldassarre 2009).

Nutrition and Exercise Important for Treating Peripheral Vascular Disease

Peripheral vascular disease involves blockage of the arteries in the legs and arms. Most patients with peripheral vascular disease are smokers, diabetics, or both. Such artery blockage can cause problems such as difficulty and pain when walking and poor healing of wounds to the hands and foot. (Please see chapter 12 for information about treating diabetic foot ulcers with good nutrition.) Peripheral vascular disease is very common in the middle-aged and elderly, with one study reporting a 19% prevalence in a group of 7,175 adults over aged 55 years (Meijer 1998).

Intermittent claudication is the most common form of peripheral vascular disease, which involves atherosclerosis-related blocking on the arteries of the legs and feet. Intermittent claudication causes pain when walking, muscle spasms, foot and leg numbness, and inability to walk for long distances. Various studies have reported that regular exercise and supplements with fish oil, 6 grams daily of L-arginine, and/or 2 grams daily of L-carnitine (amino acids), and vitamin E (400 international units or more daily) are all associated with better walking ability, blood flow, and blood vessel function in patients with peripheral vascular disease (Heffernan 2010; Carrero 2006). Other studies have reported that supplementation with ginkgo and quitting smoking can significantly reduce pain and significantly increase walking distance in intermittent claudication patients (Pittler 2005).

Any elder with symptoms of pain, numbness, or inability to walk a several blocks should consider a medical consultation to discuss testing for intermittent claudication. Inexpensive and noninvasive ultrasound tests are available to diagnose intermittent claudication and other forms of peripheral vascular disease. Many hospitals and communities also have supervised exercise programs for those with vascular problems. Smokers

LUKE CURTIS, MD

with intermittent claudication should also consider joining a smoking cessation group.

Nutrition to Lower LDL Bad Cholesterol and Triglycerides and Raise HDL Good Cholesterol

High levels of fat in the blood such as low-density lipoprotein cholesterol (also known as LDL cholesterol or "bad cholesterol") and triglycerides can greatly increase risk of many health problems including heart disease, strokes, atherosclerosis (hardening of arteries) diabetes, and even dementia (WebMD 2009; Martins 2009). Low levels of high lipoprotein cholesterol (also known as HDL or "good cholesterol") are also associated with high levels of heart disease and strokes. It is usually recommended that people keep LDL levels below 130 milligrams per 100 milliliters of blood, triglyceride levels below 150 milligrams per milliliters of blood, and HDL cholesterol levels above 40 milligrams per milliliters of blood (WebMD 2009).

About half of all seniors have high LDL cholesterol or low HDL cholesterol levels. A nationwide survey of 330 US adults over age 70 years reported that 54% had LDL ("bad") cholesterol exceeding 130 milligrams per deciliter of blood and 44% had HDL ("good") cholesterol of less than 40 milligrams per deciliter of blood (men) or less than 50 milligrams per deciliter of blood (women) (Ghandehari 2008). Lower LDL cholesterol and higher HDL in the elderly can reduce risk of heart disease, strokes, and hardening of the arteries (atherosclerosis) (Hanna 2005).

Many elders are prescribed statin drugs (such as Lipitor, Zocor, Mevacor) to lower cholesterol levels. While these statin drugs are very effective at lowering LDL cholesterol, they possess a number of bad side effects including muscle weakness and pain (especially in the legs), significantly lower coenzyme Q_{10} levels, liver problems, headaches, and digestive problems like constipation and diarrhea. Supplementation with 100 milligrams daily of coenzyme Q_{10} or more is highly recommended to all patients taking statin drugs. One New York study reported that 100 milligrams of supplemental coenzyme Q_{10} daily significantly reduced muscle pain and weakness in eighteen patients with statin-related muscle problems (Caso 2007).

Nutrition plays a key role in lowering LDL cholesterol and triglycerides and raising HDL cholesterol. Many studies have found that higher fiber consumption (especially soluble fiber from legumes and whole grains like oatmeal) are associated with a small but significant reduction in LDL cholesterol. For example, analysis of twenty-five published studies has calculated that eating a 1-ounce serving of oatmeal daily is associated with an average drop in cholesterol of about 4 milligrams per deciliter (Brown 1999). Some, but not all, studies have reported that diets containing less than 300 milligrams of cholesterol a day are associated with modestly lower blood LDL levels (Van Horn 2008).

At least ten studies have reported that regular consumption of nuts, especially walnuts, are associated with significantly lower levels of LDL cholesterol (Van Horn 2008). Analysis of thirteen published studies reported that average LDL cholesterol levels dropped by an average of 9 milligrams per 100 milliliters of blood in middle-aged and older adults consuming 1 to 2 ounces of walnuts daily (Banel 2009). All nuts are rich in omega-6 fats, minerals, fiber, vitamin E, and phytochemicals while walnuts are also very rich in omega-3 fats. Elders would be wise to consume a 1-to-2-ounce serving of nuts at least several times a week.

A number of plant-produced chemicals or phytochemicals have beneficial effects on cholesterol metabolism (Chen 2008). Phytosterols are phytochemicals, which lower LDL cholesterol. Phytosterols from pine oil are sometimes added to margarines to reduce LDL levels (Chen 2008). Such phytosterols lower cholesterol in the body by binding and excreting cholesterol in the intestines.

LUKE CURTIS, MD

LDL cholesterol may also be lowered by eating soy protein products. Soybeans contain phytoestrogens, which are similar to the human hormone estrogen. Analysis of thirty published studies has reported that eating 25 grams of soy protein per day is associated with an average reduction in blood LDL cholesterol levels of 10 milligrams per deciliter (Harland 2008). Red grapes contain polyphenols (such as resveratrol), which lower LDL and triglycerides and raise HDL cholesterol. Buckwheat contains a variety of phytochemicals, which can lower LDL and triglycerides and raise levels of HDL cholesterol. Garlic, fermented red yeast rice, and many varieties of seaweed have been shown to lower both LDL and triglycerides (Chen 2008).

Some, but not all, studies have reported that consuming yogurt and other fermented drinks containing *Lactobacillus* or *Bifidobacterium* can significantly lower LDL levels. These "probiotic" bacteria may lower cholesterol levels by absorbing and binding cholesterol in the intestine and by producing short chain fatty acids that inhibit cholesterol synthesis (Chen 2008).

The B vitamin niacin (also known as nicotinic acid) is often prescribed in large quantities (1,000 to 12,000 milligrams) to reduce "bad" LDL cholesterol and triglycerides and increase levels of "good" HDL cholesterol (Digby 2009). Some people experience skin flushing after taking niacin. To reduce risk of skin flushing, levels of supplemental niacin should be built up gradually and start at no higher than 100 to 500 milligrams daily. The author strongly urges patients with cholesterol problems to consider taking at least 200 milligrams of niacin daily. However, large quantities of niacin (over 1,000 milligrams a day) may somewhat impair blood sugar regulation. Diabetics should probably take no more than 100 or 200 milligrams of niacin daily.

Eating 4 grams or more of omega-3 fatty acids daily have also been shown to significantly reduce LDL cholesterol and triglyceride levels and significantly increase levels of HDL cholesterol (McKenney 2007). Good omega-3 sources such as fish, fish oil, flax, and flax oil should be consumed regularly by elders. For more information about sources of omega-3 fats, please see omega-3 fats section in chapter 18.

Many studies have reported that aerobic exercise has been shown to modestly reduce the levels of LDL cholesterol and modestly increase the levels of HDL cholesterol in elders (Verissimo 2002). Seniors with cholesterol problems should exercise regularly at an exercise they enjoy, such as walking, swimming, bicycling, golf, gardening, tennis, dancing, exercise class, etc.

Nutrition to Control High Blood Pressure (Hypertension)

Blood pressures higher than about 140 mm Hg systolic (systolic is the pumping phase of the heart) and 90 mm Hg diastolic (diastolic is the resting phase of the heart) can increase risk of many health problems including heart disease, strokes, diabetes, damage to vision, headaches, and dementia (eMedicine 2009; Hanna 2005). While the effects of high blood pressure (hypertension) can be devastating, the early stages of hypertension offer have no symptoms and the patient often feels fine until serious disease strikes. Since early hypertension is often silent, all adults should get their blood pressure checked at least annually.

Please note: some people get "white coat hypertension" when their blood pressure goes up about 20 mm Hg in their physicians' offices due to nervousness. People with high blood pressure in the physicians' offices should check their blood pressure in other settings such as at home or at the drugstore blood pressure machine.

A majority of elders have high blood pressure. According to the a national US survey of 2,807 adults older than 70 years, hypertension was found in 57% of white men, 69% of white women, 70% of black men, and 72% of black women. (High blood pressure was defined as blood pressure higher than 140/90 mm Hg) (Cutler 2008).

Hypertension is sometimes caused by problems with hormones, kidney malfunction, genetic problems, or birth defects such as constricted blood vessels. However, about 95% of hypertension is considered to be "essential hypertension" with no apparent cause (eMedicine 2009). In the author's opinion, most of this "essential hypertension" is due to a bad diet poor in potassium-rich fruits and vegetables. Only about one in three elders consumes the recommended daily minimum of five half-cup servings of fruits and vegetables daily (MMWR 2005). Many studies have shown that high fruit and vegetable consumption is associated with significantly lower blood pressure (Alonso 2004). More information on the link between diet and blood pressure will be presented shortly.

While nutrition plays a key role in treating blood pressure, many physicians treat blood pressure solely with a multitude of drugs and ignore nutrition. A case in point involved a 72-year-old woman with hypertension whom the author treated in medical school. This woman was generally careful with her health as she was a nonsmoker who walked 2 miles day and faithfully took four blood pressure medications daily. The four blood pressure medications she was taking included Lasix (a water removing pill), hydrochlorothiazide, Lopressor (a beta-blocker), and Lisinopril (an ACE inhibitor). In spite of taking four blood pressure medications daily, she still had high blood pressure.

The author asked how many fruits and vegetable she ate daily. She replied, "I dislike fruits and vegetables, I perhaps only eat one or two a day". He suggested the patient increase her fruit and vegetable intake. The attending doctor told him he was "crazy" to mention nutrition and merely prescribed higher levels of blood pressure medication. However the patient took his advice and her blood pressure was down 21/15 points the next time he saw her.

Good nutrition is the key to controlling most forms of high blood pressure. Limiting intake of sodium or salt is often recommended for controlling blood pressure. The average Western Diet contains about 5,000 milligrams (5 grams) of sodium daily (amounting to almost a tablespoon of salt), while only about 1,500-3,000 milligrams daily is needed to maintain health. Major amounts of salt are added to many processed foods such as soups, meats, vegetables, and many snack foods. Various studies have reported that limiting sodium intake can significantly reduce blood pressure in about half of hypertensive patients (Karppanen 2006). During the past thirty years, sodium intake in Finland has fallen by about one-third, while the average systolic and diastolic blood pressure has fallen by over 10 mm Hg, and deaths from heart disease and stroke in people under 65 years has fallen by 75% (Karppanen 2006).

Hypertensive people should consider buying lower-sodium prepared foods and add only small amounts of salt to the food they prepare. Most fresh fruits and vegetables are low in sodium, high in potassium, and are ideal for low-salt diets. Low-sodium herbal seasonings (like Mrs. Dash) can also be used to replace salt in prepared foods.

Important note: While lowering salt intake is important for hypertension patients, eating too little salt may be associated with chronic fatigue in patients with hypotension (low blood pressure). Please see chapter 15 for information on low blood pressure and chronic fatigue.

Consuming enough potassium is critical to maintaining a good blood pressure. The biggest source of potassium in the US diet comes from fruits and vegetables. As reported earlier, only a third of the elder population eats the recommended five to ten servings of fruits and vegetables daily (MMWR 2005). Bananas and citrus fruit are especially high in potassium. On the other hand, most sugary foods like colas, lemonade, and artificial fruit drinks, cookies, candy, and cake have little potassium. Numerous studies have reported that consuming higher levels of fruits and vegetables are associated with a significantly lower risk of hypertension (Alonso 2004). Various studies in developed nations have estimated that if the entire adult population consumed five or more servings a day of fruit and vegetables, hypertension rates would fall by about 50%, heart attack rates would fall by about 30%, and stroke rates would fall by 10% (Blanchard 2009).

Obtaining enough calcium and magnesium are also critical in controlling blood pressure. As noted in chapter 2, the majority of elders do not get enough calcium and magnesium in their diet. Many studies have reported that consuming low levels of calcium and magnesium are associated with an increased risk of hypertension (Karppanen 2005). Several studies have reported that taking supplements containing 1,000 milligrams or more of calcium and 400 milligrams or more of magnesium a day are associated with a significant drop in blood pressure of about 4 mm Hg systolic/2 mm Hg diastolic in hypertensive patients (Jee 2002; Van Mierlo 2006). Milk is rich in both calcium and potassium, and several studies have reported that consuming three or more glasses of milk daily is associated with significantly lower blood pressure in hypertensive patients (Kris-Etherton 2009).

Other foods and supplements may have beneficial effects on blood pressure (Chen 2009). Supplements of the amino acid L-arginine have been shown to be associated with modest declines in blood pressure. Consumption of yogurt and other fermented milk products has been associated with drops in blood pressure. This may be due to small protein products produced by the *Lactobacillus* bacteria in the yogurt. Some studies have shown that consumption of onion, garlic, and tea can modestly reduce blood pressure. Some, but not all, studies have found that consumption of soybean products can lower blood pressure. Eating Wakame (brown kelp seaweed), hawthorn, ginger, and ginkgo leaves have been associated with reduced blood pressure. The use of fish oils (rich in omega-3 fatty acids) have been associated with drops in blood pressure when consumed in high amounts (10 grams a day or more, about 2 teaspoons daily) but not at lower levels (Chen 2009).

The DASH (Dietary Approaches to Stop Hypertension) Diet has been very effective in many studies for controlling blood pressure. The DASH Diet limits sodium to 2,400 milligrams per day, includes eight to servings of fruits and vegetables daily, two servings of meat and fish, six to eight servings of whole grains, and two to four servings of low-fat milk. About half of the formerly hypertensive patients have achieved normal blood pressure on the DASH Diet (Sacks 2001). Many of these patients have also been able to reduce or eliminate their prescription blood pressure medications (Sacks 2001).

Many studies have reported that even mild to moderate exercise plays a beneficial role in reducing blood pressure in hypertensive elders (Hua 2009). Adults should pick exercise they enjoy such as walking, jogging, bicycling, swimming, golf, exercise class, dancing, weights, tennis, golf, etc. and participate for at least thirty minutes at least three times per week. Other techniques such as massage, yoga, relaxation techniques, and prayer have shown some promise in controlling hypertension.

Nutrition to Treat Asthma and Other Respiratory Disease

Asthma and other respiratory diseases are common and often under diagnosed in seniors. Among adults over age 65 years, about 5% have asthma and about 8% have emphysema or bronchitis (NIH 2009; Van Dumme 2009). Nutrition can play a major role in healing patients with many breathing diseases like asthma, emphysema and bronchitis. Good nutrition can also significantly reduce risk of pneumonia and other lung infections (please see chapter 6 for information on nutrition and infections.)

Numerous studies have reported that high consumption of fruits, vegetables are associated with lower rates of asthma and/or better-controlled asthma in both children and adults (Romieu 2001). Some, but not all, studies have reported that supplements of omega-3 containing fish or vegetable oils; vitamins B_6, B_{12}, C, E, and folate; manganese; copper; selenium; and zinc may be useful for asthmatics (Fogarty 2000). Magnesium supplements of 200 milligrams or more daily are often helpful to asthmatics (Fogarty 2000). Intravenous magnesium is often given to emergency room patients having asthma attacks and has been shown in six studies to significantly improve asthma control and reduce risk of hospitalization (Cheuk 2005). Persons with asthma and other respiratory problems should drink enough fluids, as dehydration can significantly worsen asthma and other breathing problems (Manz 2005).

Lack of protein, calories and many vitamins and minerals can have detrimental effect on patients with chronic obstructive pulmonary diseases (COPD) like emphysema and bronchitis (Berry 2001). Much more research on the effects of nutrition on COPD is needed.

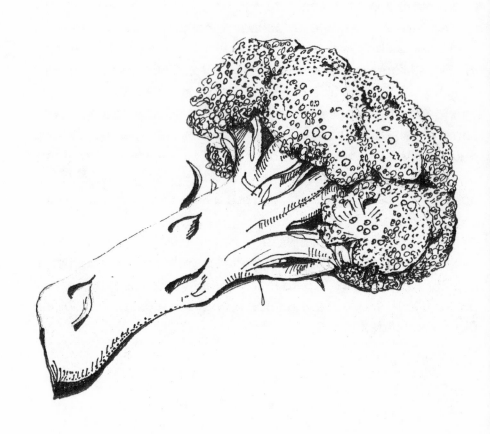

CHAPTER 9

NUTRITION TO PREVENT
AND TREAT CANCER

C ancer is one of our most feared diseases, with about 562,000 deaths annually in the USA alone (ACS 2009). More than 1 in 3 Americans are expected to develop cancer sometime in their lifetime. Most forms of cancer are much more common in the elderly than in other age groups (ACS 2009). All elders should visit their physicians at least annually and consider getting effective cancer screening tests as mammography for female breast cancer, prostate and prostate antigens tests for prostate cancer, and colonoscopy to test for intestinal cancers. Smoking is also a major risk factor for many cancers including those of the lung, breast, prostate, and many other organs. Please see chapter 8 for tips on quitting smoking.

Much research has found that good nutrition can significantly prevent many types of cancer. Some recent research has also found that good nutrition can also improve survival and/or reduce cancer recurrence in patients who already have cancer.

Nutrition to Prevent Cancer

Many studies have reported that diet may play a role in preventing cancer (Milner 2002; Donaldson 2004; Divisi 2006). Many, but not all, studies have indicated that adequate consumption (in food or supplements) of items such as fruits and vegetables (especially berries and vegetables from the cruciferous [broccoli, cabbage] and allium [onion, garlic] families); fiber; omega-3 fatty acids; probiotics; carotene; selenium; vitamins B_{12}, C, D; and folate are associated with lower incidence of many types of cancer (Milner 2002; Donaldson 2004; Divisi 2006).

Hundreds of studies have reported that high consumption of fruits and vegetables (more than about 5 or 6 half-cup servings daily) are associated with much lower rates of cancer incidence. A review of 170 published studies reported that 132 studies (78%) found that high fruit and vegetable consumption significantly reduced cancer incidence, while only 6 studies (4%) were associated with a significantly higher cancer rate was associated with high fruit and vegetable intake (Block 1992). High fruit and vegetable consumption was protective in 24 of 25 studies (96%) for lung cancer; 28 of 29 studies (97%) of mouth, throat, and esophagus cancer; 20 of 27 (74%) studies of cancer of the colon and rectum; 3 of 5 studies (60%) of bladder cancer; 10 of 12 studies (83%) of cancers of the cervix, uterus, and ovaries; and 8 of 14 studies (57%) of breast cancer (Block 1992). Many of these studies also reported that higher consumption of beta-carotene (a form of vitamin A found in yellow and green vegetables like carrots, pumpkin, sweet potatoes, broccoli, spinach, and parsley) was associated with significantly lower rates of many different kinds of cancer. Consumption of a related phytochemical called beta-cryptoxanthin has been associated with significantly lower rates of breast and lung cancer (Gallicchio 2008). Beta-cryptoxanthin is found in a wide range of vegetables

LUKE CURTIS, MD

including peppers (especially red peppers), cilantro, parsley, papayas, oranges, and watermelon.

Fruit and vegetable consumption was least protective of prostate cancer, with only 4 of 14 studies (28%) showing a significant protective effect of high produce consumption (Block 1992). However, 6 out of 8 studies have reported that consuming lycopene (a red phytochemical contained in tomatoes and watermelon) is associated with significantly lower rates of prostate cancer (Haseen 2009). The author consumes tomatoes or tomato juice daily to protect against prostate cancer. Lycopene is also available in supplement pills.

Broccoli and Other Cruciferous Vegetables Reduce Risk of Many Cancers

Cruciferous vegetables include broccoli, cauliflower, brussels sprouts, kale, cabbage, bok choy, and radish. Cruciferous vegetables are so named since they have cross shaped flowers. Cruciferous vegetables are rich in many vitamins (especially vitamins A and C), minerals, and helpful phytochemicals such as sulforaphane. Sulforaphane has strong cancer-fighting properties and also helps boost the immune system and control blood sugar in diabetics. Sulforaphane is found in especially high levels in broccoli and broccoli sprouts. Both human and animals studies report that regular consumption of cruciferous vegetables can reduce risk of many cancers (Clarke 2008).

Cruciferous vegetables may be especially helpful for preventing lung cancer. Lung cancer is the deadliest form of cancer, which kills about 160,000 in the United States annually (Medicine Net 2010). A recent California study compared consumption of dietary isothiocyanates (found mostly in cruciferous vegetables) in 311 lung cancer cases and 622 controls. Lung cancer rates were only 65% as high among subjects consuming four or more servings of cruciferous vegetables weekly as compared to subjects consuming less than one serving a week of cruciferous vegetables. These results were statistically significant and were adjusted for exposure to active and secondhand smoking (Carpenter 2009). The author urges all seniors to consume at least four to seven servings of cruciferous vegetables every week.

Many Fruits and Vegetables Reduce Risk of Cancer

Berries contain many vitamins and a wide range of phytochemicals (such as polyphenols, lignans, flavonoids, and triterpenoids), which have cancer-fighting properties. All of the commonly eaten berries such as blueberries, raspberries, blackberries, cranberries, strawberries, pomegranate, and acai berries are rich in phytonutrients. Many studies with lab animals and cell cultures have reported that berries have strong anticancer properties. A preliminary human study has found that daily consumption of 45 grams of black raspberries may reduce esophageal cancer risk in patients with a premalignant condition called Barrett's esophagus (Seeram 2008). Pomegranate and pomegranate juice shows considerable promise in fighting many cancers such as breast and prostate (Heber 2008). Citrus fruits such as oranges, grapefruits, lemons, and limes contain significant amounts of flavonoid phytochemicals, which have significant anticancer properties in studies with lab animals and cell cultures (Benavente-Garcia 2008).

Resveratrol is a phytochemical found in red/purple grapes, berries, and peanuts. Many animal and cell culture studies have reported that resveratrol has major benefits in both preventing cancer and slowing aging by reducing cell oxidation damage. Several human studies are currently underway to see if resveratrol reduces incidence of human cancers (Udenigwe 2008).

Another group of vegetables with probable anticancer properties is the Allium family, which includes garlic, onions, leeks, and chives. These vegetables contain several sulfur-containing phytochemicals (such as allicin and diallyl sulfide), which have both strong anticancer and anti-infective properties. Daily consumption of high levels of garlic (10 or more grams daily) was associated with significantly lower rates of cancers of the stomach, esophagus, and colon in 6 out of 11 (54%) human studies (Shukla 2007).

Soybeans are rich in high-quality protein, unsaturated oil, calcium, iron, and phytochemicals called isoflavones. These isoflavones mimic the activity of the hormone estrogen. Some studies have linked consumption of 25 more grams a day of soybean protein to lower levels of cancers of the breast, endometrium, and prostate (McCue 2004). Many women with family histories of breast cancer consume soy products daily to probably reduce their risk of getting breast cancer. Soybeans can be eaten in many forms, including as tofu curd, miso paste, roasted soy nuts, baked soybeans, soy flour, soy grits, and isolated soy protein. The author especially enjoys adding soy grits to cereals, breads, and meat dishes.

The relationship between fat intake and breast cancer has been extensively studied. Higher levels of omega-3 fat consumption, relative to consumption of omega-6 and saturated fat consumption, has been linked to significantly lower rates of breast cancer (Duncan 2004). Other studies have reported that consumption of 2 tablespoons or more of olive oil daily is associated with significantly lower rates of breast cancer (Duncan 2004). Olive oil is rich in monosaturated fats but does not contain a high level of omega-3 and omega-6 unsaturated fats. Some, but not all, studies have linked obesity and high total fat intakes to higher rates of breast cancer (Duncan 2004).

Vitamin D, Selenium, Zinc, and Other Supplements Reduce Cancer Risk

Some, but not all, studies report that vitamin D and other dietary supplements reduce cancer risk. As noted in chapter 2, vitamin D deficiency is very common in elders, with about 76% of US whites and 96% of US blacks over the age of 60 years having low blood vitamin D levels (Ginde 2009). A number of studies have reported that higher consumption of vitamin D (from diet, supplements, or sunshine) is associated with lower rates of colon, prostate, breast, mouth, and ovarian cancer as well as leukemia (Donaldson 2004). Some researchers estimate that US colon cancer incidence could be reduced by 50% and US breast cancer rates could be reduced by about 30% if all adults obtained adequate vitamin D levels by taking 2,000 international units of supplemental vitamin D daily (Garland 2007).

Some studies have reported that higher consumption of folate and/or vitamin B_{12} (in food or supplements) is associated with significantly lower rates of breast and colon cancer (Donaldson 2004; Martinez 2006). A huge study of 35,242 middle-aged and elderly men reported that supplementation with 15 milligrams of zinc daily was associated with significantly lowered rates of advanced prostate cancer (Gonzalez 2009). Consumption of folate and vitamin C have been linked in some, but not all, studies to significantly lower rates of breast cancer (Duncan 2004). Supplementation with 200 micrograms daily of selenium daily has been associated with significantly lower rates of cancers of the prostate, rectum, and colon (Donaldson 2004).

Nutrition to Treat Cancer and Cancer-Related Malnutrition

Malnutrition is very common in cancer patients. About 30 to 85% of all cancer patients experience malnutrition, significant loss of lean body tissue, and cancer-related loss of appetite (cachexia) (Argiles 2005). Cancer-related malnutrition is especially common in patients with pancreatic, stomach, esophageal, head/neck, lung, and colon cancers (Argiles 2005).

Many studies have noted that cancer-related malnutrition and weight loss causes considerable morbidity and mortality (Argiles 2003). A study of 3,047 cancer patients found that survival rates in patients with 5% or more weight loss was significantly lower in nine out of twelve types of cancer (Dewys 1980). This same study reported that among 290 patients with favorable non-Hodgkins lymphoma, five-year survival rates were 90% (179/199) among patients who had not lost more than 5% of their weight, but only 33% (30/91) among patients who lost more than 5% of their pre-lymphoma weight (results were very statistically significant) (Dewys 1980).

Most cancer patients are advised to eat a well-balanced diet with lots of water, fruits, vegetables and whole grains, moderate amounts of lean meat, fish, eggs, dairy products, nuts, and legumes and low levels of saturated/trans fats, refined sugars, and alcohol (Doyle 2006). Some cancer patients cannot get adequate nutrition via the oral route and must receive some or all of their nutrition via tube feeding (Argiles 2005; Doyle 2006). (For more information on tube feeding, please see chapter 7). Many cancer patients will benefit by consultation with a dietician or other nutritional expert (Doyle 2006).

What specific types of foods and supplements seem particularly helpful to cancer patients? As noted earlier, many studies relate nutrition to cancer prevention, but relatively few studies have examined the effects of diet on survival and cancer relapse rates in patients who already have cancer. Preliminary research has indicated that a diet rich in omega-3 fatty acids (especially EPA), antioxidant vitamins, and polyphenols (found in grapes, green tea, and other fruits/vegetables) may be useful in the limiting the inflammation and weight loss caused by cancer-related loss in appetite (McCarthy 2003). Supplements of proteins and/or amino acids may also be helpful to cancer patients who have lost lean weight. A study of patients with solid tumors and significant weight loss found that the use of a supplement containing arginine, glutamine, and beta-hydroxy-beta-methylbutyrate (HMB) significantly increased body mass relative to placebo (May 2002).

A study of 65 bladder cancer patients noted a 41% five-year tumor recurrence rate among patients given a vitamin and zinc supplement with megadoses of vitamin A, B_6, C, E and zinc as compared to a 91% tumor recurrence rate among patients given a supplement with only the US Recommended Daily Allowance (RDA) of vitamins and zinc (Lamm 1994). A Japanese study reported that oral supplements of Lactobacillus casei significantly reduced recurrence of superficial bladder cancer (Aso 1995). A study of 442 patients with non-small-cell lung cancer found that higher blood levels of vitamin D levels were associated with a 55% lower death rate (Zhou 2007). Higher consumption of dry beans and fish were associated with significantly lower rates of colon cancer recurrence, while higher consumption of vitamin D, folate, and calcium supplements was associated with slightly lower rates of colon cancer recurrence (Mathew 2004; Hartman 2005; Lanza 2006). A prospective study of 1,009 patients with stage III colon cancer found that adherence to a Western diet containing high amounts of meat, fat, refined grains, and desert was associated with a significantly higher death rate and cancer recurrence as compared to a "prudent diet", which emphasized vegetables, fruits, fish, and poultry (Meyerhardt 2007). Note: all seven of these studies mentioned in this paragraph produced results, which were very statistically significant.

While it is clear that a diet rich in fruits and vegetables can reduce the incidence of some cancers, it is less clear whether or not such a diet can improve survival or reduce tumor recurrence in cancer patients. An Australian study of 609 women with invasive epithelial ovarian cancer reported that higher consumption of vegetables was associated with a 25% lower mortality rate and higher consumption of cruciferous vegetables (such as broccoli and cabbage) was also associated with a 25% lower mortality rate (Nagle 2002). However, other large studies with breast cancer and lung cancer patients have reported that high consumption of vegetables are associated with only small and nonsignificant declines in death rates (Skuladottir 2006; Pierce 2007). Women with breast cancer who had higher serum levels of carotenoids (carotenoids are found in many vegetables like carrots) had a significantly longer period of disease-free survival (Rock 2005). Consumption of higher levels of tomato sauce and fish were associated with lower rates of prostate cancer recurrence (Chan 2006).

In the future, large, well-controlled studies are needed to develop better nutritional treatment regimes for patients with cancer. Further study of nutritional effects of cancer will need to account for many factors like type and stage of cancer, types of treatment used (chemotherapy, radiation, surgery), genetics, and noncancer health problems of patients.

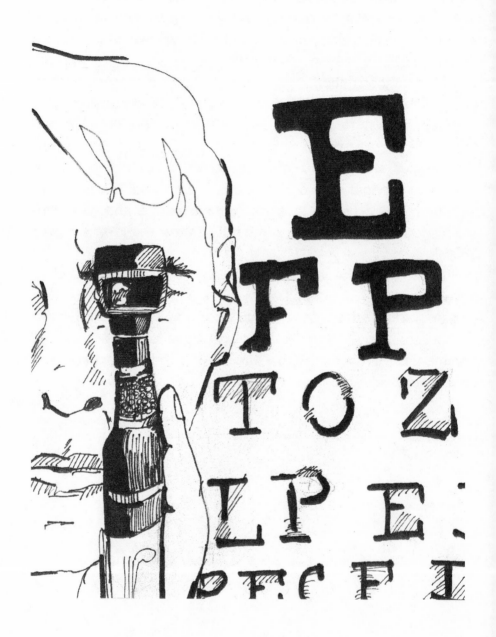

CHAPTER 10

NUTRITION TO IMPROVE EYESIGHT

F ailing eyesight is common among seniors. The author has treated many seniors who were active and generally healthy but whose quality of life was greatly diminished by falling eyesight. Poor eyesight makes common activities like reading, walking, and driving difficult or impossible. Poor eyesight also increases risk of falls, depression, and social isolation (Pelletier 2009). He remembers his grandmother who lived to be 98 years old in good health until about age 95 years, except that she was limited by poor eyesight.

The most common cause of vision problems in seniors is macular degeneration, which affects about 10% of the population between 65 and 74 years, 30% of the population between 75 and 84 years and 50% of the population over 85 years old (Eye Digest 2009). Macular degeneration involves damage to the nerve cells in the back of eye or retina. The macula is a nerve-rich area in the back of the eye that converts chemical signals into electrical signals that are sent to the brain. Macular degeneration patients often have severely worsened sight in the center of the field of vision, but milder vision loss on the edges (periphery) of their vision. Severe macular degeneration can lead to persons becoming blind or nearly blind.

Another common cause of loss of vision in elders is cataracts, which involve darkening of the lens of the eye. Most people over 65 years have at least mild cataracts on one of both of their lens, while cataracts sufficient to significantly impair vision are found in about 10% of those older than 65 years (Wrong Diagnosis 2009).

Damage to the retina in the back of the eye (diabetic retinopathy) can also cause substantial vision loss. Diabetic retinopathy causes damage to the blood vessels in the eye. Good control of blood sugar can greatly reduce risk diabetic retinopathy in diabetics (Cheng 2009). Diabetes should aim for a fasting blood sugar level of less than 120 milligrams per 100 milliliters of blood or a hemoglobin A1C level of less than 5.5-6.0% (Cheng 2009). (Please also see chapter 12 for more on information on the control of blood sugar and hemoglobin A1C in diabetics). Glaucoma or excessive pressure in the eye can also cause visual impairments in the older age group.

All persons older than 65 years should receive a thorough eye exam at least every one to two years. Persons experiencing sudden vision loss should contact a physician immediately, as this could indicate a sight-threatening condition such as acute glaucoma. Seniors may also need new eyeglass prescriptions every one to three years.

A Good Diet and Supplements Are Critical for Maintaining Eye Health in Seniors

While eye problems are common in the elder years, good nutrition can play a major role in preventing or slowing down progression of these eye problems. A number of studies have reported that diets/supplements containing high in fruits, vegetables, vitamins C and E, beta-carotene (a form of vitamin A found in yellow vegetables like carrots and pumpkin), zinc, and copper was associated with significant slowing of the progression of age-related macular degeneration (AREDS 2001). Diets high in omega-3 fatty acids and/or fatty fish/fish oils are also associated with significantly lower incidence of macular degeneration (SanGiovani 2008). Another large study reports that diets high in the phytochemicals lutein and zeaxathin were also associated with significantly lower rates of macular degeneration (Tan 2008). Lutein and zeaxathin are found in many vegetables such as corn, kale, broccoli, turnip and collard greens, spinach, zucchini, and watermelon. Lutein is also found in egg yolks.

An interesting study from the Czech Republic reported that nutritional supplementation may not only slow progression of macular degeneration but may actually help reverse the effects. This study reported that year-long daily supplementation with 200 milligrams of acetyl-N-carnitine (an amino acid), 20 milligrams of coenzyme Q_{10}, and 4 grams of omega-3 fatty acid-rich fish oil significantly improved vision in macular degeneration patients, while no vision improvement was seen in macular degeneration patients given placebo (Feher 2005).

A number of studies have also suggested that consuming diets high in fruits, vegetables, whole grains, and fish may slow cataract progression (Moeller 2004). Other studies have reported that supplements with B complex vitamins such as thiamin (B_1) and riboflavin (B_2) and vitamin E may also slow progression of cataracts (Jacques 2005).

Both a good diet and proper supplementation are crucial for maintaining eye health. The Age-Related Eye Disease Study Group (AREDS) is a consortium of scientists in New Zealand, Australia, United States, and Britain who are studying eye health. They recommend consuming food supplement(s) containing at least the following levels of nutrients daily (Raniga 2009). Note that one tablet of many multivitamin mineral supplements do not contain enough of these nutrients.

1. Beta-carotene, 15 milligrams (which is equal to 25,000 international units of vitamin A)
2. Vitamin C, 500 milligrams
3. Vitamin E, 400 international units
4. Zinc 80, milligrams
5. Copper, 2 milligrams

To protect their eyesight, the author recommends that all seniors consume at least five half-cup servings of a wide range of fruits and vegetables daily, and fish at least twice a week. Eating dark green and yellow vegetables like carrots, pumpkin, sweet potatoes, broccoli, parsley, dandelion greens, leaf lettuce, spinach, and mustard or collard greens are especially important since these vegetables are rich in "phytochemicals" such as lutein and beta-carotene. Elders should also consume supplements containing vitamin B complex, C and E, zinc, copper, L-carnitine or acetyl-N-carnitine (amino acids), and coenzyme Q_{10}. All of these supplements are available without a prescription. Prices of supplements vary greatly, so be sure to shop around stores and the Internet for best prices.

Protect Your Eyesight by Wearing UV Blocking Sunglasses and Not Smoking

Elders should also protect their eyes by wearing UV-blocking sunglasses in the sun and by not smoking. Studies show that wearing such UV light-resistant sunglasses throughout the lifespan can reduce risk of macular degeneration (Delcourt 2001) and cataracts (Neale 2003) in the elderly.

Not smoking or quitting smoking is also important to maintain eye health. Various studies have reported that smoking increases risk of macular degeneration (Coleman 2009) and cataracts (Linblad 2005) in the elderly. Other studies report that exposure to secondhand tobacco smoke, wood burning smoke, and air pollution may increase risk of macular degeneration and cataracts (Pokhrel 2005).

Proper control of blood sugar through diet and exercise is also critical for maintaining eye health in diabetics. Please see tips for controlling diabetes in chapter 12, "Nutrition to Prevent and Treat Diabetes".

Nutrition to Improve Night Vision

Some seniors have trouble with night vision. Many seniors have told the author that they have no trouble driving during the day but cannot drive at night due to night vision problems. Troubles with night vision can be caused by cataracts (clouding of the eye lens) or by problems of the retina (the retina is the back of the eye and gathers light and processes it into nerve signals to send to the brain). Nutritional factors to prevent or slow cataract formation have been discussed earlier in this chapter. Many nutrients have been proven to be helpful for night vision. Patients deficient in vitamin A suffer night vision problems since their retinal cells cannot make sufficient chemicals called rhodopsin in order to detect light and color (Sklan 1987). The author has seen several vitamin A deficient seniors improve their night vision significantly after being given a better diet with supplements of beta-carotene. As mentioned above, vitamins C and E, zinc, and copper are critical for maintaining retinal health needed for good night vision. Phytochemicals such as lutein from green vegetables are also important for eye health.

Some researchers believe that eating bilberries (*Vacinnium myrtillus*) or bilberry jam improves night vision due to the anthocyanoside phytochemicals they contain. During World War II, British pilots were given bilberry jam several hours before they went out on night missions. Research on bilberries and night vision has been mixed, with some studies indicated that bilberries are helpful for night vision and other studies showing they have little effect on night vision (Canter 2004).

Better nutrition can greatly improve eyesight. One patient of the author was a 91-year-old lady who was in generally good health except she could not see well due to advanced macular degeneration. She could not read regular-sized print or even walk very well due to her limited eyesight. Her diet was fairly good, except that she ate only about three servings of fruits and vegetables daily. She followed the author's suggesting of upping her fruit and vegetable intake up to at least five servings a day. At his suggestion, every day she also took an eye multivitamin and mineral supplement with 1,000 milligrams of vitamin C, 400 international units of vitamin E, 80 milligrams of zinc, and 2 milligrams of copper. In addition, she also took 1 tablespoon of cod-liver oil, 100 milligrams of coenzyme Q_{10}, and 1,000 milligrams (1 gram) of L-carnitine daily. Following a year of such diet change, her vision improved to the point where should could read regular-sized print (12 point), work on her stamp collection, and engage in several activities at her church. Consultation with her eye doctor (ophthalmologist) revealed that her macular degeneration regressed considerably following a year of better diet and supplements.

LUKE CURTIS, MD

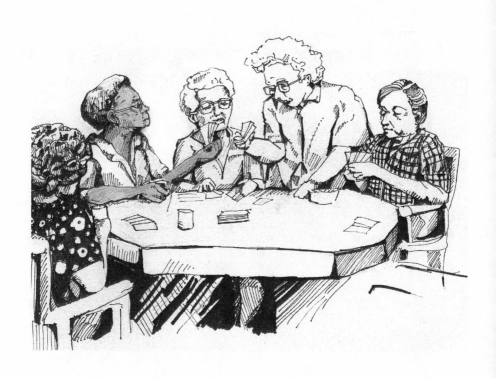

CHAPTER 11

NUTRITION TO PREVENT AND TREAT DEMENTIA, DEPRESSION, AND HEADACHES

Nutritional Treatments to Prevent or Slow Alzheimer's and Other Dementias

Perhaps the most feared health problem of older folks is dementia. Dementia patients have severe declines in their mental abilities, lose a lot of muscle weight, and often require assistance for such basic activities such as eating, bathing, and dressing. Oftentimes they cannot even recognize family members. While the most common form of dementia is Alzheimer's disease, many other conditions can cause dementia including strokes; traumatic brain injury; brain infections (HIV, syphilis); advanced Parkinson's disease; alcohol or drug abuse; nutritional deficiencies (such as low vitamins B_1 [thiamine], B_{12} [cobalamin], folate, and niacin); thyroid problems; Lewy bodies (abnormal proteins that collect in nerve cells); and many genetic diseases. Alzheimer's disease is an all too common disease found in about 0.3% of US 70-year-olds, 1.4% of 80-year-olds and 5.9% of 90-year-olds (Brookmeyer 1998).

The good news is that good nutrition can play a role in slowing down or even preventing the development of Alzheimer's and other dementias. Omega-3 fats are critical to brain health but are low in most US diets. An Illinois study of adults older than 65 years reported that consumption of fish once or more per week was associated with a 60% lower risk of development of Alzheimer's as compared to those who rarely ate fish (Morris 2003). Similar studies conducted in France and Japan have also concluded that moderate consumption of fish and other sources of omega-3 fats were associated in significantly lower rates of Alzheimer's as compared to those who consume little omega-3 fats. A Swedish study of 204 patients with early Alzheimer's reported that daily supplementation with 4 grams of fish oil in one year resulted in significantly better appetite and weight gain as compared to placebo receiving corn oil capsules (Irving 2009).

Although consumption of omega-3 fats may be protective against Alzheimer's, several studies have reported that high consumption of either saturated fats or trans fats are associated with significantly higher rates of Alzheimer's disease (Morris 2009). Saturated fats are found primarily in fatty meat and dairy products. Trans fats are food in many fried foods (such as fast-food french fries), donuts and other baked goods, and in some margarine and in peanut butter prepared with hydrogenated oil.

A number of studies with older humans have reported that eating five or more fruits and vegetables daily significantly reduces risk of developing Alzheimer's disease and similar forms of dementia (Hughes 2009). Animal studies have reported that consumption of blueberries, red or purple grapes or grape juice, pomegranates, and walnuts provide considerable protection against the development of Alzheimer's (Joseph 2003 and 2006; Hartman 2006). All four of these foods are rich in plant produced phytochemicals, while walnuts are also fairly high in omega-3 fats.

LUKE CURTIS, MD

Some recent studies have reported that daily consumption of either blueberry juice or Concord grape juice can improve mental function in elderly humans. In Ohio, a group studied the effects of consuming either about half a liter (a little more than a pint) of blueberry juice or a non-juice-containing placebo beverage. The subjects were over 70 years of age (average age 76 years), in good general health but with some memory decline. After twelve weeks, several forms of memory were significantly improved in the nine subjects receiving the blueberry juice but memory remained unchanged in the seven subjects given placebo (Krikorian 2010). A similar study reported that consumption of half a liter of Concord grape juice for twelve weeks significantly improved memory in older adults, while those who consumed a placebo beverage had no improvement in memory (Krikorian 2009). Both blueberries and Concord grapes are rich in phytochemicals, which may improve and preserve mental function. Eating the whole blueberry or Concord grape fruits would probably also result in memory gains.

Some, but not all, studies have reported that consumption of the antioxidant vitamins C and E are associated with lower risk of Alzheimer's disease. A Dutch study of 5,395 adults over age 55 years reported that consumption of moderately high levels of vitamin C and E (in the diet or supplements) was associated with about a 40% lower risk of getting Alzheimer's disease (Engelhardt 2002). Another study reported that lower blood vitamin D levels were associated with significantly worse mental function in Alzheimer's patients (Oudshoorn 2008).

Deficiencies in magnesium, zinc, and many of the B vitamins such as thiamine (B_1), riboflavin (B_2), pyridoxine (B_6), folate, and vitamin B_{12} can also cause dementia and related neurological problems in the elderly (Balk 2006). As noted in chapter 2, deficiencies in vitamin B_{12} are very common in the elderly with one large study reporting that 40.5% of seniors over the age of 67 years are vitamin B_{12} deficient (Lindenbaum 1994). Vitamin B_{12}

deficiency can cause many problems including lack of red blood cells (anemia), dementia, chronic fatigue, many neurological problems, and depression. Supplementation with vitamin B_{12} and other B vitamins can cause dramatic improvement in mental abilities, energy levels, mood, and neurological symptoms in those who are deficient in vitamin B_{12}.

The author has seen several vitamin B complex deficient demented elder patients improve dramatically in a matter of weeks when give supplements of B complex vitamins.

Nutrition to Prevent or Treat Depression in the Elderly

Depression is also very common in elders, occurring in about 20% of community living seniors and 20-45% of those in elder care facilities (Jones 2003; Grunebaum 2008). As with dementia, nutrition plays a key role in preventing or treating elder depression. A number of studies have linked deficiencies in protein, calories, and other nutrients to higher rates of depression in the elderly (Smoliner 2009).

A good general diet may reduce risk of depression. A French study of 1,724 adults over age 65 years reported that high consumption of fruits, vegetables, and fish were associated with significantly better mental function and less depression (Samieri 2008).

Consumption of omega-3 fats from fish, fish oil, flax, and other sources can significantly reduce risk of elder depression. Analysis of ten double-blind studies reported that supplementation with 1 or more grams of omega-3 fatty acids per day were associated with a large and significant reduction in adult depression (Lin 2007). (A double-blind study is a study where neither the researchers nor the subjects know who is given the active nutrient and who is given the placebo). Most, but not all studies of seniors over 65 years have also reported that consumption of fatty fish or omega-3 rich oils are associated with significantly lower rates of depression. For example, a Greek study of 1,190 adults over age 65 years found that consumption of fatty fish once or more per week was associated with a 58% reduced risk of depression compared to the seniors who did not consume fish (Bountziouka 2009). For more information about sources of omega-3 fats, please see omega-3 fats section in chapter 18.

Besides omega-3 fats, many other nutrients play a role in preventing depression. Lack of many nutrients such as protein, calories, omega-3 fats, magnesium, zinc, and vitamin C and many B vitamins are associated with depression in adults (Larson 1992). Providing proper amounts of these nutrients in the diet/ supplements can often improve depression. Several studies on depressed adults have reported that 500 to 5,000 micrograms (0.5 to 5 milligrams) daily of folate can be useful in improving symptoms in depressed adults (Sarris 2009). Other studies have reported that supplementation with 800 to 1,600 milligrams a day of the amino acid S-adenosylmethionine (SAMe) significantly reduced depression in adults (Alpert 2004). A number of studies have reported that the use of herb St. John's wort (*Hypericum perforatum*) is helpful to patients with mild depression (Miller 1998).

Depressed patients have a lack of a brain chemical called serotonin in the spaces or junctions between the nerve cells. The amino acid 5-hydroxy tryptophan is a building block to synthesize serotonin in the body. Providing the body with supplements of the amino acid tryptophan or 5-hydroxy tryptophan can increase levels of serotonin the nerve cell junctions and help to relieve depression. Analysis of eleven published studies has reported that of 451 depressed patients who took 50 to 600 milligrams daily of supplemental 5-hydroxy tryptophan daily, 244 or 54 % had their depression significantly reduced (Turner 2006). 5-hydroxy-tryptophan is now available as a food supplement in vitamin and health food stores. Milk, beef, turkey, chicken, and fish are also very rich in the amino acid tryptophan and are sometimes recommended for depressed patients to help rebuild their supplies of serotonin.

A good diet and broad-based supplementation is a good way to fight senior depression. A study of 225 hospitalized patients over age 65 years gave them a liquid supplement containing the recommended dietary intakes for many vitamins and minerals or a placebo containing few nutrients. After six months' treatment, the elders receiving the vitamin-mineral supplement had significantly lower rates of depression than the group who received the placebo (Gariballa 2007). Many nutrients such as omega-3 fats, B vitamins, zinc, and magnesium are also often useful for patients with chronic fatigue or fibromyalgia (please see chapter 15).

Avoiding Toxins Is Important to Prevent Depression and Dementia

For good mental health, seniors should also try to reduce their exposures to common chemical toxins. Exposure to many chemicals such as pesticides (Stallones 2002), lead (Golub 2009), and molds and their mycotoxins (Shenassa 2007) have also been associated with high levels of mental depression and even to significantly higher suicide rates. Some, but not all studies have linked smoking and exposures to aluminum, arsenic, mercury, and pesticides to higher levels of dementia (Dosunmu 2007).

Elders who live in homes/apartments built before the 1970s should consider getting their homes evaluated for lead paint, as lead paint was commonly used in US homes before the 1970s. Spraying of pesticides should be avoided in indoor environments or less toxic insect control alternatives should be used such as boric acid or pesticide traps. Any signs of visible mold growth or water leaks in homes should be cleaned immediately or dangerous levels of molds and mycotoxins can quickly build up.

Physical and Mental Exercising Also Crucial in Preventing Depression and Dementia

Exercise is especially useful for battling depression in elders. A review of eleven published studies involving elders reported that moderate exercise, such as walking or exercise class twenty to sixty minutes three or more times per week is associated with significantly lower levels of depression (Blake 2009). Exercise is helpful for depression in a number of ways. It increases the levels of hormones called endorphins in the body. Endorphins give a feeling of well-being, euphoria, and a sort of "natural high". Exercise also improves blood flow to the brain and other parts of the body. In addition, exercise is often done with other people and promotes social bonding.

As mentioned before, it is important for elders to pick an exercise they enjoy so they will stick within for the long run. Walking, bicycling (standard or stationary bike), swimming, dance, exercise class, golf, and tennis are all excellent exercises for seniors. Having an exercise partner joining an exercise group or fitness club/YMCA can also encourage elders to continue regular exercise.

Several studies have reported that physical exercise like walking, exercise class, or gardening are useful in slowing or preventing dementia (Perez 2008; Galluci 2009). A combination of good diet, supplements, mental and physical exercise, and avoidance of toxic chemicals may provide the best way of lowering risk of dementia. A study of 1,880 older adults in New York City reported that adults who exercise and consume a Mediterranean Diet (rich in vegetables, fruits, whole grains, fish, and olive oil) have a significantly lower risk of getting Alzheimer's and depression (Scarmeas 2009).

While physical exercise can help to prevent or slow dementia, mental exercise can also keep mental skills sharp and prevent or at least slow the onset of dementia. Various studies of adults aged 70 to 100 years have reported that reading daily for a half hour or more, solving sudoku or crossword puzzles, playing bridge, and getting regular social contact and conversion are all associated with significantly less mental decline with age and significantly lower risk of getting Alzheimer's dementia (Galluci 2009; Clarkson-Smith 1990; Times Online 2005). Mental functions are the same as physical functions in that they usually age much slower when provided with exercise. "Use it or lose it" applies to both physical and mental functions.

Religious Support Can Also Reduce Risk of Depression and Dementia

Belonging to a religious group, prayer, yoga, and meditation can reduce risk of both depression and dementia. Hundreds of worldwide studies have reported that belonging to a religious group can greatly reduce risk of depression in the elderly (Koenig 2009). One huge Utah study of 2,989 adults between the ages of 65 to 100 years reported that those who attended church three or more times per month had only about half the rate of depression of those who attended church less than once per month (Norton 2008). A few studies have also reported that regular attendance at religious services is associated with lower levels of dementia and mental decline in older adults (Reyes-Ortiz 2009). The author encourages all elders to join or continue their involvement in religious communities for the social and religious support they provide.

Nutrition Can Also Help Control Headaches

While headaches are somewhat less common in older adults than younger adults, they are still very common with about 10% of women and 5% of men reported bad headaches at least monthly (Reinisch 2008). Any elder with prolonged or severe

LUKE CURTIS, MD

headaches should consult a physician to rule out a more serious problem like a stroke or brain tumor. However, the vast majorities of headaches are not life threatening but are very annoying and can adversely affect work and sleep.

Dietary factors can often influence headaches. Skipping meals or eating huge meals are associated with higher risk of headaches (Millichap 2003). Allergies to many foods such as chocolate, cheese, milk, grain, soybeans, and peanuts have been associated with headaches (Millichap 2003). Any elder who regularly develops headaches after eating a certain food should consider getting tested for food allergies. Another common trigger for both headaches and asthma is monosodium glutamate (MSG) (Toth 2003). About 2% of the US population is sensitive to MSG. MSG-related adverse reactions are often hard to diagnose since MSG-related headaches and asthma can take up to twenty-four hours after eating the MSG to develop. The author advises all patients to avoid MSG as much as possible. MSG is commonly added to many foodstuffs such as meats, fish, and Chinese foods. When dining out in a Chinese restaurant, always request that the food be prepared without MSG.

Supplements can be helpful to chronic headache patients. Various studies have reported that treating patients with 400 milligrams or more a day of magnesium is often helpful in reducing migraine headaches (Biondi 2003). The use of intravenous (i.e., injected into a vein) magnesium is often used in hospitals to stop severe headaches. Some studies have reported that daily supplementation with 300 milligrams of coenzyme Q_{10}, 1 tablespoon or more of fish oil, and high dose vitamin B complex supplements are associated with significantly fewer and milder headaches (Sandor 2003; Biondi 2003). A Brazilian study reported that 3 milligrams of melatonin at bedtime was associated with total or major reduction in 78% of a group of 32 migraine headache patients (Peres 2002). (Please see chapter 15 for more information on melatonin and sleep).

Headaches can be triggered by many common chemical exposures such as pesticides, perfumes, formaldehyde, paints, secondhand tobacco smoke, and molds (Martin 1993). Many elders have reported relief for headaches after reducing their exposures to common toxic chemicals. Regular exercise and sexual intercourse can also be helpful to elders with chronic headaches. One study of forty women with chronic headaches found that regular aerobic exercise (such as brisk walking) reduced headache symptoms by about 55% (Narin 2003). Another study of fifty-seven women reported that sexual intercourse relieved headaches in 47% of patients, caused no change in headaches in 47%, and worsened headaches in only 6% (Evans 2001).

LUKE CURTIS, MD

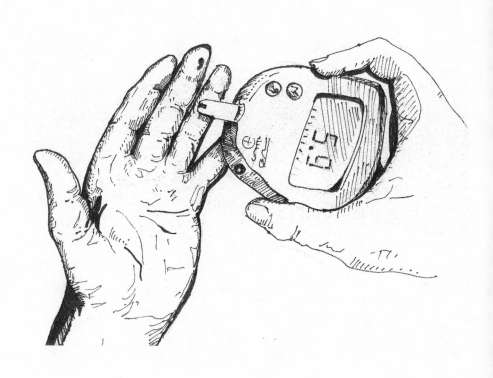

CHAPTER 12

NUTRITION TO PREVENT
AND TREAT DIABETES

Diabetes is very common in elders with about 10% of those over age 65 having diabetes (Chau 2001). There are two types of diabetes: type 1 or juvenile diabetes and type 2 or adult-onset diabetes. Type 1 diabetes involves autoimmune destruction of the beta-cells in the pancreas, which produce insulin. Insulin is a hormone that plays a central role in controlling levels of sugar in the blood. A type 1 diabetic must take insulin daily for the rest of their life. Type 1 diabetes usually begins in children or young adults who are underweight or normal weight. In type 2 diabetes, the body develops resistance to the insulin the pancreas produces. Such insulin resistance causes blood sugar to rise.

Type 2 diabetics usually begins in overweight older adults, although type 2 diabetes can also occur in teenagers and/or thin people. Most type 2 diabetics can be treated with diet and oral diabetic medication, although some type 2 diabetics require insulin. About 95% of diabetes is type 2 (WebMD 2009).

Many people with type 1 and type 2 diabetes lead healthy and productive lives. The author knows of many diabetic patients who work full-time jobs and engage in endurance exercise such as marathon running (26.2 miles) or century bike riding (100 miles). However, diabetes puts a person at greater risk for many health problems, including heart disease, strokes, kidney problems, hardening of the arteries (atherosclerosis), poor wound healing, vision problems, problems in *Candida* overgrowth, and erectile dysfunction in men (WebMD 2009).

Blood sugar control is measured by two methods: (1) levels of the sugar glucose in the blood and (2) levels of hemoglobin A1C in the blood. All diabetes should get their blood sugar monitored daily and their hemoglobin A1C levels measured at least every three months. Blood sugar is usually measured by fasting eight or more hours. Fasting blood sugar levels above 120 milligrams per 100 milliliters of blood indicate the patient probably have diabetes and requires further testing. Levels of hemoglobin A1C is a measure of the number of hemoglobin molecules in the blood that have had sugar molecules added on. (Hemoglobin is the molecule in the blood that transports oxygen and carbon dioxide and gives blood its red color.) Higher levels of sugar in the blood produce higher hemoglobin A1C levels. Since hemoglobin has a life span of three months in the blood, the hemoglobin A1C levels is a reflection of blood sugar levels over the past three months. Diabetics or persons at risk of getting diabetics should aim for a hemoglobin A1C level of not higher than 7.0% (Chau 2001). A number of studies have reported that keeping hemoglobin A1C levels below 7.0% can greatly reduce risk of diabetic-related health problems such as heart disease, kidney failure, and strokes (Khaw 2006).

It is critical that diabetics measure and control their blood sugar carefully. If blood sugar becomes very high, diabetes can go into diabetic ketoacidosis. If the blood sugar becomes too low, they can go into diabetic coma. Both diabetic ketoacidosis and diabetic coma can be life threatening. Diabetics and people at risk for diabetes should measure their blood sugar regularly.

Many convenient automatic blood sugar monitors are available. Blood monitors are under development, which does not require a skin prick for a blood sample (Chu 2008). Diabetics should also receive regular physician visits and take their insulin and/or other diabetic medications regularly. Diabetics should always carry snacks containing both protein and carbohydrates at all times in case their blood sugar drops.

Diet Is the Cornerstone for Avoiding or Controlling Diabetes

While medication, physician visits, and regular monitoring of blood sugar are critical in diabetes, diet plays the most important role in avoiding or managing diabetes. Weight control is also critical for diabetes as being overweight or very underweight can greatly worsen the problems associated with diabetes.

The cornerstone of prevention of obesity and type 2 diabetes is a well-balanced diet of at least three meals a day containing a mixture of protein, carbohydrates, and fats. It is crucial that diabetics eat regularly and often and not skip meals or eat huge meals. Meal skipping has been associated with much poorer blood sugar control in diabetics (Rost 1990). High-protein snacks like milk or yogurt or a small serving of cheese, meat, or nuts should be eaten as between-meal snacks to keep blood sugar levels high. A well-balanced vitamin/mineral supplement containing calcium, magnesium, zinc, chromium, and B vitamins is also a good idea for diabetics.

Each meal should contain a protein source such as lean meat/poultry, fish/shellfish, eggs, milk/yogurt, or low-fat cheese like cottage cheese. The daily diet should provide at least five half-cup servings of fruits and vegetables, preferably prepared without added fats and sugars. Alcohol and refined sugars such as cane sugar, corn syrup, and honey should be avoided. Refined grains like white flour and white rice should also be avoided.

Eating a diet containing at least 25 grams of fiber may also be useful in controlling diabetes. Fiber-rich foods include most fruits and vegetables (not juices), nuts and seeds, and whole grains. Fruit and vegetable juices are not good sources of fiber since most of the fiber has been removed. Most of the fiber has been removed from fruit juices. Some studies have shown that daily consumption of five servings or more of fruits and vegetables are associated with modestly lower rates of new onset type 2 diabetes in middle-aged or older adults (Liu 2004). Some, but not all studies have reported that diets high in fiber are useful for controlling both excess weight and diabetes (Nahas 2009). Other studies have reported that higher consumption of whole grains and/or lower consumption of refined sugar are related to significantly lower risk of adults over age 55 years developing type 2 diabetes (Meyer 2000).

Consumption of peanuts and tree nuts can also be helpful in preventing and treating diabetes. One study reported that consumption of 5 ounces or more weekly of nuts, peanuts or peanut butter was associated with a significantly lower risk of getting type 2 diabetes in middle-aged women (Jiang 2002). Another study reported that feeding adults 30 grams of nuts daily (a mixture of walnuts, almonds, and hazelnuts) was associated with significantly better blood sugar control in patients with type 2 diabetes (Casas-Agustench 2009).

Elders are often deficient in chromium (Vaquero 2002). Chromium is needed to make a protein called glucose tolerance factor that helps to control diabetes. Many studies have reported that low chromium is associated with higher risk of type 2 diabetes (Vaquero 2002). A number of studies have reported that taking 200 micrograms daily of supplemental chromium is useful for controlling diabetes (Nahas 2009).

Many foods are now being tested for the presence of plant-based chemicals or "phytochemicals", which play a role in preventing or controlling diabetes. Foods that contain phytochemicals show promise in controlling blood sugar in diabetics including soybeans, broccoli, onions, sweet potatoes, cinnamon, blueberry and many other fruits, vegetables, and herbs (McCue 2005; Sheela 1995; Ludvik 2008; Suppapitiporn 2006; Martineau 2006; Li 2004). Much more research on the effects of phytochemicals on the effects of diabetes is needed.

The causes of type 1 diabetes are not fully known. However, it has been shown in many studies that consumption of supplemental vitamin D can significantly reduce the risk of developing type 1 diabetes and other autoimmune diseases like lupus (Stechschulte 2009). The author recommends that all adults who do not receive considerable sun exposure consume at least 800 international units of vitamin D in their diet and supplements.

Exercise and Proper Weight Crucial for Controlling Diabetes

Many studies have reported that regular exercise is associated with lower weight, better blood sugar control, and low levels of LDL cholesterol in diabetes (Magkos 2009). Be sure to pick an activity you enjoy such as walking/jogging, bicycling, swimming, dancing, exercise class, weight lifting, golf, tennis, gardening/yard work, or even vigorous play with children/grandchildren/dogs. Having an exercise partner or joining a walking, biking, dance, or exercise group is often helpful for people needing to lose weight. Many elders exercise regularly with a dog, spouse, boyfriend/girlfriend, sibling, parent, neighbor, or coworker.

To lose weight, try to exercise at least one hour at a time at least three to five times per week. To burn the maximum number of calories, it is better to exercise longer at a moderate pace that exercise intensively for short periods. For example, it is best to walk, jog, bike, stationary bike, or swim at a moderate pace for a half hour to hour or so than to run, bike, or swim all out for a few minutes at a time and then become quickly exhausted.

Slow weight loss is best; it is best not to lose more than 1 or 2 pounds of weight per week. Faster weight loss often leads to health problems such as chronic fatigue, weakness, depression, constipation, and increase susceptibility to illness. Near-starvation diets lower a person's metabolic rate as the body tries to save energy and go into a famine mode. Following a starvation diet, persons tend to regain weight quickly since their metabolism has been lowered by a too-low calorie diet (Mole 1990).

It is critical that patients with diabetes or at risk of diabetes avoid or at least limit intake of concentrated sugar sources such as refined sugar, corn syrup, honey, molasses, and dried fruit. To provide sweetness to foods, try using fresh fruit or natural low-calorie sweeteners like Stevia. Stevia powder is made from the leaves of several related shrubs that grow in South America and is about 300 times as sweet as ordinary table sugar (sucrose). Stevia has been enjoyed for hundreds of years and has also no reported adverse side effects in hundreds of published reports (Goyal 2009). Stevia powder packets are available for sale in most health food stores and large supermarkets. Many of the author's friends and family have enjoyed using Stevia as a sweetener. Other low-calorie sweeteners include aspartame (which consists of phenylalanine, aspartate, and a methyl group); sucralose (a sugar molecule with three chlorine atoms added); and acesulfame-K (Whitney 2008).

Diabetic patients are more likely to suffer eye problems like glaucoma, macular degeneration, and damage to eye blood vessels (diabetic retinopathy) as compared to nondiabetics. All diabetics should see an eye doctor (ophthalmologist or optometrist) at least once a year. For information on nutritional approaches to preventing or slowing eye disease, please see chapter 10.

LUKE CURTIS, MD

Better Nutrition and Faster Diabetic Wound Healing

Diabetics often suffer from delayed wound healing. The most common wound healing problems involve ulcers of the feet, ankles, or abdomen. These skin ulcers are painful and may become infected. Good nutrition can do much to speed up wound healing in diabetic and other patients. A great many nutrients are required for wound healing including fluids, protein (especially the amino acid arginine), omega-3 fats, zinc, iron, copper, magnesium, selenium, chromium, and vitamins A, B complex, C, E, and K (Ord 2007). Many of these nutrients are deficient in most diabetic patients. Eating a good diet and receiving vitamin/ mineral and arginine supplements can often speed up wound healing in diabetics. One study reported that supplying elderly diabetic patients with pressure ulcers a liquid dietary drink rich in protein, arginine, vitamin C, and zinc double the rate of ulcer healing (Cereda 2009).

Nutrition can have a dramatic effect on healing even large and infected diabetic wounds. The author treated one man with diabetes with four large infected abdominal wounds that ranged in size from a golf ball to a baseball. He had these wounds chronically for over a year. The author suggested he eat a well-balanced diet plus a vitamin and mineral supplement, extra iron and zinc, omega-3 from fish oil, and Juven amino acid supplement (which consists of glutamine, arginine, and leucine). After three months of better nutrition, the four large wounds were almost completely healed!

Wound Care Clinics Also Very Helpful in Healing Chronic Wounds

In addition to excellent nutrition, the author urges that all patients with large or persistent diabetic wounds/ulcers should visit a wound care clinic to take advantage of many of the latest treatment advances. Several studies have reported that treatment in a specialized wound clinic is associated with much better rates of wound healing and much lower rates of amputation as compared to standard care (Sumpio 2004). He has seen many diabetic patients whose feet were so badly infected that amputation was suggested. After several months of excellent nutrition and wound clinic care, their feet were almost completely healed and many returned back to work full-time!

To reduce risk of foot problems, all diabetics should wear comfortable, well-fitted shoes and receive foot exams from a physician at least once a year.

LUKE CURTIS, MD

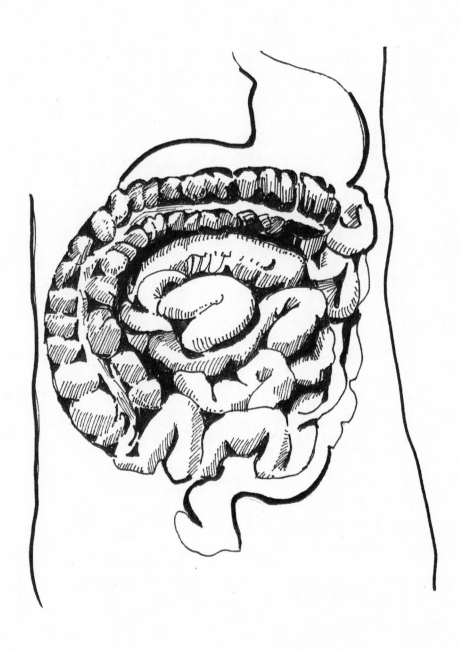

CHAPTER 13

NUTRITION TO PREVENT
AND TREAT DIGESTIVE PROBLEMS

D igestive problems are common in elders. In US adults over age 65 years, the prevalence of heartburn is about 10-20%, discomfort from stomach or intestinal ulcers about 9%, and presence of irritable bowel syndromes is about 6-18% (Crane 2007). About 15% of the population over age 80 years have a moderate to severe case of diverticulitis (diverticulitis involves formation of pockets in the colon) (Salzman 2005). Irritable bowel syndrome and diverticulitis are somewhat overlapping disorders, which can cause abdominal pain, bloating, constipation, and diarrhea. All of these digestive disorders make eating uncomfortable and may cause significant reduction in food intake and malnutrition.

Treatment of Heartburn and Ulcers

Heartburn or esophageal reflux involves food from the stomach being passed upward through the esophagus. Prolonged heartburn greatly increases risk of esophageal cancer.

Eating meals quickly and/or eating large meals increases risk of heartburn. Eating three or more small- to moderate-sized meals can greatly reduce the risk of heartburn symptoms. Eating slowly and chewing food carefully can also reduce risk of diverticulitis. Also, heartburn-prone elders should avoid eating or lying down within one hour of eating to allow their food to pass through their stomach. Severe cases of heartburn require medical examination and possible surgery (Heidelbaugh 2003).

Ulcers involve tissue damage to the stomach of upper intestine or duodenum. They frequently cause a great deal of pain and discomfort. At one time, ulcers were thought to be caused by psychological factors like worry. Now we know that most ulcers are caused either by bacteria called *Helicobacter* or by use of nonsteroidal anti-inflammatory drugs (NSAIDS) like aspirin, ibuprofen, and naproxen. These NSAIDS erode the surface of the stomach and intestinal walls. Anyone suspecting ulcers should contact a physician. Most ulcers can be controlled by a combination of antibiotics and a proton pump inhibitor medicine like Prilosec, Prevacid, or Nexium. NSAIDS-related ulcers can generally be treated by either discontinuing the medication or by taking coated NSAIDS (such as coated aspirin) with meals (Ramakrishnan 2007).

Some dietary factors can also help prevent ulcer formation. Consumption of omega-3 fats and probiotic bacteria such as *Lactobacillus* are associated with faster healing of stomach and intestinal ulcers. Eating various phytochemical-rich foods such as Korean red ginseng, green tea, purple grapes, garlic, broccoli sprouts, and cranberries also inhibit *Helicobacter* growth in the stomach (Lee 2008).

LUKE CURTIS, MD

Treatment of Bloating, Abdominal Pain, Diarrhea, and Constipation

Many elders with digestive problems are prescribed medications like laxatives and antidiarrheal medications to treat bloating, diarrhea, and constipation. While these medications may provide short-term relief, a good diet is the cornerstone for restoring the gut to long-term health.

Mild causes of irritable bowel syndrome (IBS), diverticulitis, and chronic diarrhea or constipation can often be treated with diet. IBS patients are urged to consume a well-balanced diet with sufficient liquids and plenty of fiber including lots of fruits and vegetables (Mayo Clinic 2009). Sweets, alcohol, fruit juices, and refined grain products (like white rice and white bread) should be avoided on an IBS diet. Whole fruits and whole grains contain much more fiber than their fruit juice and refined grain counterparts. All food eaten should be fresh, as rotten food can be filled with bacteria and toxins from bacteria (Mayo Clinic 2009). Moderate exercise and sufficient sleep can also help the digestive process.

The use of fiber from psyllium seeds (such as Metamucil) is often recommended for persons with constipation. A British study of 275 patients with irritable bowel syndrome treated patients with either 10 grams of psyllium fiber or 10 grams of wheat bran fiber or 10 grams of placebo white rice flour. About half of these patients had diarrhea predominant IBS and about half have constipation dominant IBS. The patients receiving the psyllium fiber treated had significantly less diarrhea, constipation, and abdominal pain as compared IBS patients given either bran or placebo. The water soluble fiber in the psyllium may be more helpful to treating irritable bowel syndrome than the water insoluble fiber in the bran (Bijkerk 2009). Psyllium must always be consumed with sufficient liquids such as water, milk, or juice.

Other studies have reported that the soluble fiber found in soybeans, other beans like navy and kidney beans, and oatmeal are especially good for treating problems of constipation, diverticulitis, and irritable bowel (Bennett 1996). Eating apples is good for treating mild diarrhea since apples are rich in pectin, and pectin tends to produce well-formed stools. Many studies have reported that eating plums and prunes are associated with fewer problems with constipation, diverticulitis, and irritable bowel. Plums and prunes are a good gentle cure for constipation since they are rich in both fiber and a sugar called sorbitol that has mild laxative effects (Stacewicz 2001). For maximum benefit, all fiber-rich foods need to be consumed with adequate liquids.

Persons with irritable bowel syndrome or chronic diarrhea may also benefit from supplements of partially digested whey protein, partially digestive short chain fatty acids, and digestive enzyme supplements (Cook 1998; Yalcin 2006). Digestive enzyme supplements contain enzymes found in gut to digest proteins (proteases like pepsin), fats (lipases), and carbohydrates (cellulases, lactase, maltase, sucrase) in the gut. Partially digested whey protein, partially digested fats, and digestive enzymes are available at health food stores without a prescription.

Probiotic bacteria like *Lactobacillus* and *Bifidobacterium* can also help reduce the symptoms of abdominal pain, diarrhea, and constipation in irritable bowel patients. A review of eight randomized, placebo-controlled trials reported that use of probiotic bacteria significantly reduced the diarrhea, constipation, and abdominal pain common in IBS (Nikfar 2008). Probiotic bacteria are also frequently included in tube feeds to patients being given enteral (tube) nutrition (DeLegge 2008). (Please see chapter 7 for information on tube-feeding patients.)

Probiotic bacteria may also be helpful in chronic constipation as well. A review of five recent studies with chronic constipation patients have reported that use of probiotic bacteria such as *Lactobacillus casei*, *Bifidobacterium lactis*, and *Escherichia coli* were associated with more frequency bowel movements, better bowel movement consistency, and less discomfort as compared

LUKE CURTIS, MD

to patients given placebo (Chmielewska 2010). Much more research is needed to find the best probiotic strains to treat irritable bowel syndrome and other health problems.

Consumption of probiotic bacteria or yogurt containing probiotics may also reduce the risk of bacterial and yeast infections in areas outside the digestive tract. A New York study of thirty-three women with repeated vaginal infections of Candida (a mold or yeast) reported that daily consumption of yogurt containing live (viable) acidophilus cultures cut rates of vaginal Candida infection by about 80% (Hilton 1992).

For a free copy of an article the author wrote on irritable bowel syndrome, please contact him at LukeTCurtis@aol.com.

Note: Patients with severe or prolonged symptoms of diarrhea, constipation, or blood in the stools should consult a physician in order to rule out more serious conditions like colon cancer, ulcerative colitis, or Crohn's disease.

Food Allergies May Also Cause Problems for the Digestive and Other Systems

Food allergies are common in elders, with one recent study reporting that 25% of a group of 109 elders (aged 60 to 94 years) had one or more food allergies (Bakos 2006). Food allergies such as gluten allergy (celiac disease) may also cause moderate to severe digestive discomfort in elders. Food allergies can cause many symptoms including irritable bowel like bouts of diarrhea and constipation, asthma, skin rashes, headaches, and mental confusion. Anyone who suspects a food allergy should consult a physician about possible skin prick or blood testing for food allergies. After allergic patients stop eating the foods they are allergic to, their health will often significantly improve. A Kansas study of 20 middle-aged and older adults with irritable bowel syndrome reported that their symptoms of pain, diarrhea, and constipation significantly improved after they eliminated the foods they were allergic to. Patients were also given a daily probiotic supplement containing 10 billion *Lactobacillus*, *Bifidobacterium*, and *Streptococcus* bacteria (Drisko 2006).

A particularly bad form of food allergy is celiac disease or gluten allergen. Celiac disease is present in about 1% of adults over age 60 years, although a majority of celiac patients are undiagnosed (Rashtak 2009). Celiac disease can cause many problems including diarrhea, constipation, abdominal pain, asthma, skin rashes, headaches, and mental problems. The diarrhea produced by celiac disease may lead to lack of many nutrients, especially fat soluble vitamins like vitamins A, D, and E (Rashtak 2009).

Several blood tests, such as the antiendomysial test, are available in physicians' offices to diagnose celiac disease. Once diagnosed, celiac disease patients can often improve greatly if they carefully avoid all gluten-containing products. Wheat, rye, barley, spelt, teff, and triticale all contain gluten and must be avoided. Oats do not contain gluten but contain a related protein, which some celiac patients are allergic to. Celiac patients need to read food labels to check for all sources of wheat and other gluten containing grains. For whole grains, celiac patients can eat cereals or breads made from rice, wild rice, corn (including popcorn), millet, buckwheat, and amaranth (Rashtak 2009).

Even small amounts of gluten can be harmful to celiac patients. Several case reports have been made about celiac patients reacting to the small amount of gluten found in wheat communion wafers! If requested, most churches will gladly prepare communion wafers prepared with a nongluten grain such as rice or corn (Groce 2008).

The author strongly urges that all patients with digestive problems such as diarrhea and constipation or problems like asthma, headaches, or confusion get tested for food allergies, including allergy to gluten.

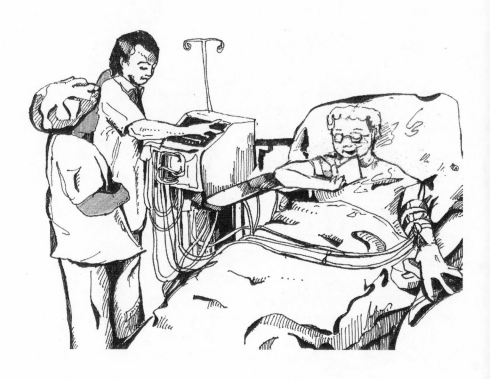

CHAPTER 14

NUTRITION TO PREVENT
AND TREAT KIDNEY FAILURE

The kidneys are two remarkable organs that filter about 1,700 liters or 1,900 quarts of blood daily (Berne 1998). The kidneys play a critical role in removing toxins, waste, and water from the body.

One can live well with only one kidney, provided the kidney is working well (Berne 1998). However, kidney problems can sometimes develop for a variety of reasons including genetics, infection, toxic chemicals or drugs, diabetes, or removal of one kidney from cancer. About 0.7% of US adults over age 65 years are in severe kidney failure, while an additional 4.5% of elders have lower kidney function that has the possibility of developing into kidney failure (Arora 2009).

Avoiding Kidney Failure

The best way to treat kidney failure is prevention. A good diet can substantially cut the risk of developing kidney failure in the first place. The two most common causes of kidney failure are high blood pressure (hypertension) and diabetes (Snyder 2005).

Eating a well-balanced diet with protein at least three times daily, at least five servings of fruits and vegetables daily and limiting consumption of sugar and refined grains can do much to avoid both high blood pressure and diabetes. For more information about nutritional prevention/treatment of high blood pressure, please see chapter 8, "Nutrition to Treat Heart, Vascular and Lung Problems". For more information about nutritional prevention and treatment of diabetes, please see chapter 12, "Nutrition to Prevent and Treat Diabetes".

Other nutritional factors can prevent kidney disease. Several studies have reported that adequate blood levels of vitamin D and/or vitamin D supplementation can significantly slow rates of kidney failure development (Melamed 2009). Supplementation or high dietary intakes of B vitamins such as folate, B_6 (pyridoxine), and B_{12} (cobalamin) can also reduce kidney failure development by reducing blood levels of a toxic protein called homocysteine (Clements 2006). Patients at risk for kidney disease should consume about 1 gram of protein per kilogram of body weight per day. For a table of protein content in common foods, please see the protein section in chapter 18. Eating a diet either very low or very high in protein can increase risk for kidney failure (Clements 2006).

Various drugs like analgesics (aspirin, Tylenol, Motrin, Alleve, etc.), many antibiotics, many chemotherapy drugs and statin drugs (used to treat high levels of blood fats and include such common drugs as Lipitor, Pravachol, Crestor, and Zocor) can also damage kidneys and increase risk of kidney failure (Naughton 2008). Toxic chemicals like lead, mercury, ethylene glycol (found in antifreeze), and some toxins from molds (mycotoxins) like ochratoxins can also damage the kidneys (Naughton 2008). Smoking also greatly increases risk of kidney failure (Clements 2006).

What to Do if Kidney Failure Occurs

Kidney failure is a serious problem involved in many possible complications, including significantly higher death rates. The author is not trying to minimize the difficulties associated with kidney failure. However, he has seen many patients with failed kidneys live decent lives when given dialysis or kidney transplantation and excellent nutrition.

Kidney failure can be treated either with dialysis or by kidney transplantation. Dialysis can involve hemodialysis in which a patient goes to a dialysis center three times a week for several hours to get their blood filtered. Peritoneal dialysis involves surgically placing a bag in the patients' abdomen, which filters blood, by the use of a salt-containing solution. Kidney transplantation involves transplanting a kidney from a living or dead donor.

While kidney dialysis is certainly unpleasant, many dialysis patients can still have a decent quality of life. The author met one interesting 83-year-old man who developed kidney failure and was on dialysis for the past five years. Despite being on kidney dialysis, the man mentioned he was still working twenty to forty hours a week and walking 2 miles a day for exercise. He was still quite active in his church, did some traveling with his wife, involved with his grandchildren, and still having regular sex with his wife. This man was an immigrant from Italy who later served in the US navy at the end of world war. After dating several girlfriends, he finally married, had three children, and ran a grocery store. At 65, he went to college for the first time in his life to obtain a BS in computer engineering in just three years. For the past fifteen years, he has been working on repairing computers.

Kidney transplants are often effective even in patients older than age 70 years (Heldal 2009). Older kidney failure patients may have a lower priority on kidney transplant lists, but can often get a kidney donated from a relative or friend. The author saw one 71-year-old HIV-positive gentleman who did well after receiving a kidney from his 21-year-old granddaughter. Now he is working part-time, walking 2 miles daily, and attending White Sox and Cubs games in person.

Diet and Supplements for Kidney Dialysis Patients

Kidney dialysis patients have complicated nutritional needs. They need to consume appropriate amounts of water and minerals such as sodium, potassium, phosphorus, calcium, and magnesium. Kidney failure patients should get the advice and direction of a nutritionist, nurse, or physician knowledgeable about nutrition for kidney patients. A complete discussion of all of the management issues of dialysis patients is beyond the scope of this book.

Dialysis patients should eat at least three well-balanced meals of meat, fish, eggs, dairy products, whole grains, fruits, and vegetables. Some dialysis patients may have to limit their intake of certain nutritious foods in order to limit their intake of water, sodium, potassium, and phosphorus. For example, a patient who has high levels of potassium may need to limit intake of high-potassium foods like tomatoes, potatoes, bananas, and citrus fruit.

Dialysis patients are often malnourished due to poor diet and loss of vitamins, minerals, and amino acids via dialysis (Sen 2000). Various published studies have reported that from 31% to 92% of hemodialysis patients are seriously deficient in the following nutrients: protein; calories; carnitine; coenzyme Q_{10}; zinc; vitamins D, C, B_1 (thiamine), B_{12} (cobalamin); and folate (Cianciaruso 1995; Perunicic 2007; Debska 2007; Triolo 1994; Cabral 2005; LaClair 2005; Hung 2001; Chadna 1997; Bamonti 1999; Fehrman-Ekholm 2008). Dialysis patients should design an individualized supplement program with the help of a nutritionist or nutrition minded physician or nurse.

LUKE CURTIS, MD

Protein balance is especially critical for renal patients. Too little dietary protein causes excessive breakdown of body protein, while too much protein can put excessive stress on kidneys (Kopple 2001). Meta-analysis of twelve studies found that restricting protein in diabetic renal patients (most of them not on dialysis) to 0.7 to 1.1 grams/kilogram bodyweight/day was associated with a slowing of progression of kidney failure (Robertson 2007). For a more table of protein content in common foods, please see the protein section in chapter 18.

Overall nutritional status and nutritional supplementation may play an important role in reducing morbidity and mortality in dialysis patients. A study of fifty-five patients on chronic hemodialysis found that the estimated death risk was nine times as great in patients who had moderate or severe malnutrition as compared to well-nourished patients (Cusumano 1996). Supplementation of omega-3 fatty acids in dialysis patients has been found to significantly increase hemoglobin and albumin, significantly reduce inflammation, and significantly reduce risk of heart attack rates (Perunicic 2007; Friedman 2006; Svensson 2006). Supplemental L-carnitine has been found to have many beneficial effects on dialysis patients, including better red blood cell production, less inflammation, more protein production, better heart function, and improved blood sugar control (Guarnieri 2007). A double-blind placebo-controlled study of twenty-one chronic dialysis patients found that patients given 180 mg coenzyme Q_{10} daily had significantly less need for dialysis and significantly higher blood antioxidants levels as compared to patients given placebo (Singh 2000). A study of 51,037 hemodialysis patients found that mortality was cut 48% in patients taking injected supplemental vitamin D ($p < 0.001$) (Teng 2005).

While dialysis patients may often benefit from nutritional supplementation, excessive amounts of nutritional supplements may be harmful to dialysis patients since reduced kidney function may lead to harmful buildup of water soluble vitamins, minerals, and amino acids in the body. Of special concern is vitamin C. Dialysis patients are often very low in vitamin C since they can lose several hundred milligrams of vitamin C in each dialysis session (Handelman 2007). However, excessive vitamin C can cause toxic buildup of oxalate in bloodstream and kidneys (Handelman 2007). Intake of up to 500 mg a day of vitamin C by dialysis patients is believed to be safe (Keven 2003). A recent study of hemodialysis patients reported that consumption of 200 milligrams of supplemental vitamin C daily was associated with prevented vitamin C deficiency in nearly all dialysis patients without producing a toxic buildup of vitamin C or oxalate (Fehrman-Ekholm 2008).

Dialysis patients often have chronic low levels of red blood cells (anemia). They are sometimes given a drug called erythropoietin to increase red blood cells levels. Studies with anemic hemodialysis patients have found that erythropoietin is effective in increasing red blood cells only if the diet contains adequate levels of protein, calories, copper, iron, folate, carnitine, and vitamins C and E (Akgul 2007; Higuchi 2006; Johnson 2007).

A sensible diet and moderate amounts of supplements seems to be best for dialysis patients. In the future, comprehensive nutritional testing of blood and other tissues may lead to better development of individualized nutritional regimes for dialysis patients. More research on nutrition for renal patients is needed in order to determine both positive and negative effects of specific diets and nutritional supplements

LUKE CURTIS, MD

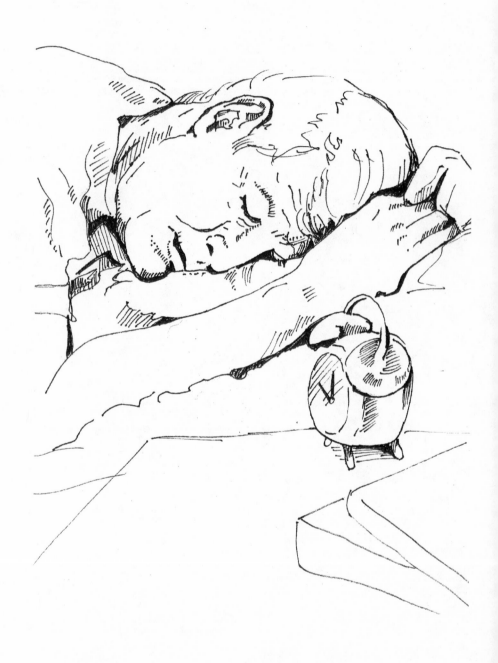

CHAPTER 15

NUTRITION TO TREAT CHRONIC FATIGUE, FIBROMYALGIA, AND SLEEP PROBLEMS SUCH AS SLEEP APNEA

M any elders feel tired all of the time. Chronic fatigue is often considered just a part of growing old. Various surveys have reported that roughly 20-50% of adults over age 70 years report moderate to severe fatigue all or most of the time (Wick 2007; Tralongo 2003). Some seniors also have fibromyalgia, a condition of chronic fatigue coupled with joint problems. A French study of 1,014 adults reported that 2.8% of adults of ages 65 to 74 and 4.1% of adults from 75 to 84 met criteria for fibromyalgia (Bannwarth 2009).

Most people of all ages experience considerable fatigue after losing sleep, after getting a mild infection like a cold, or after a heavy bout of work or exercise. However, severe fatigue all of the time usually indicates some health problems such as nutritional deficiencies, sleep apnea, thyroid problems, anemia (deficiency of red blood cells), chronic infections such as *Candida* or Lyme disease, cancer, severe depression, or heavy exposure to mold and chemicals. In many cases, these chronic fatigue-producing conditions can be effectively treated and the seniors' energy and vigor restored.

Nutritional Strategies to Treat Chronic Fatigue and Fibromyalgia

Many nutritional problems can cause chronic fatigue. Probably the most common fatigue causing nutritional problem in the elderly is anemia, or a low red blood cell count. Lack of red blood cells can hinder the body's ability to bring oxygen to the cells and remove carbon dioxide. About 10% of the US population over 65 years suffers from anemia (Guralnik 2005). As noted in chapter 2, many elders' diets are deficient in nutrients needed to make blood in the bone marrow, including protein, calories, iron, zinc, copper, folate, and vitamins B_6 and B_{12}. Improved diet and proper supplements can oftentimes greatly improve red blood count in elders (Guralnik 2005). Elders with chronic anemia should consult with their physician to rule out non-nutritional cases for anemia such as cancer.

Note: Many kidney failure patients have anemia and chronic fatigue, which can be helped by proper diet and supplements. Please see chapter 14 for nutritional guidelines for kidney failure patients.

Getting enough protein and calories is important to maintain good energy levels. As noted in chapter 2, at least 16% of community living elders and 42-91% of hospitalized elders do not get enough protein or calories. Protein-calorie malnutrition can lead to loss of muscle (sarcopenia), bone (osteoporosis), and significantly lower energy levels (Theou 2008). Not getting enough liquids can also cause dehydration, which can also lead to many problems including fatigue, dry skin, and heart, lung, blood vessel, and circulatory problems. As noted earlier, elders should consume at least six 8-ounces glasses of liquid daily

LUKE CURTIS, MD

and eat at least 1 gram of protein per kilogram (2.2 pounds) of bodyweight.

Many nutrients play a role in facilitating the body's energy-producing reactions and fighting fatigue. The B vitamins play a major role in many of the body's energy-producing and tissue-building reactions. A number of studies have reported that chronic fatigue patients are often low in vitamin C and B vitamins such as B_1 (thiamine), B_2 (riboflavin), B_6 (pyridoxine), B_{12} (cobalamin), and folate and often benefit from supplementation (Werbach 2000). Magnesium is a mineral that plays a role in over five hundred of the body's metabolic reaction and is often low in chronic fatigue patients. One study reported that daily supplementation with 300 milligrams of magnesium and 1,200 milligrams of malic acid significantly reduced pain and fatigue in twenty-four fibromyalgia patients (Russell 1995). Malic acid is a molecule involved in the body's energy production cycles. Chronic fatigue patients are also often low in zinc and may benefit from supplementation (Werbach 2000).

Too Little Sodium (Salt) in the Diet
Can Cause Chronic Fatigue

Surprisingly enough, many chronic fatigue and fibromyalgia patients are low in sodium. Lack of sodium may cause low blood pressure (hypotension). This hypotension is often especially bad just as a person is getting up from lying down in bed (this is called "orthostatic hypotension"). Many of these patients are lacking in sodium after following low-sodium diets recommended by the media and physicians. One study of twenty-three chronic fatigue patients reported that twenty-two (96%) had orthostatic hypotension. Most of these patients had been following a low-salt (sodium) diet. Following a diet with adequate amounts of water and sodium, nine of the patients (39%) had complete or near complete resolution of their fatigue. Some of these patients also received the medication fludrocortisone to help increase their blood pressure (Bou-Holaigah 1995).

The author recommends that all chronic fatigue and fibromyalgia patients receive and continue taking regular amounts of sodium in their diet, unless they have high blood pressure or kidney problems or advised otherwise by their physicians. He also recommends that all elders measure their blood pressure at least once every three months. Both low and high blood pressure carries significant health risks to elders. (For information on controlling *high* blood pressure through better nutrition, please see chapter 8). Many pharmacies have automatic blood pressure cuffs in which patrons can monitor their blood pressure at no charge.

Iodine deficiency can also cause thyroid problems, which can cause chronic fatigue. A recent survey of human iodine levels in the USA reported that 6.7% of US adults over age 70 years are deficient in iodine (Caldwell 2008).

Iodine is essential for essential thyroid function and energy production. The best sources of iodine include saltwater fish and shellfish, sea vegetables like kelp and dulse, iodized salt and iodine supplements. Whole grains and vegetables grown on iodine-rich soil are also fair sources of iodine. People on low-sodium diets may have to limit their intake of salt and sea vegetables, which are high in sodium as well as iodine. (More information on sea vegetables is provided in chapter 17, "Near-Ideal Diets").

As noted in chapter 2, most people of all ages are not getting enough omega-3 fats in their diet. Omega-3 fats play a key role in reducing inflammation and fighting chronic infections that can cause chronic fatigue. Fish and flax oil supplementation can improve symptoms in chronic fatigue patients. A double-blind study of sixty-three patients with postviral fatigue gave patients 8-500 milligrams capsules of either an omega-3-rich fish and evening primrose oil mixture or olive oil. Following three months

LUKE CURTIS, MD

of treatment, fatigue symptoms improved significantly in 85% of the patients given the fish/primrose oil mixture but improved in only 17% of the patients given olive oil (Behan 1990).

Two nutrients, which are often low in chronic fatigue patients, are coenzyme Q_{10} and carnitine. Coenzyme Q_{10} is a vitamin-like substance that plays a major role in metabolic processes that produce energy for the body. Coenzyme Q_{10} can be synthesized by the body, but its synthesis can be blocked in people taking statin drugs (such as Lipitor, Pravachol, Crestor, Zocor) for high cholesterol. Coenzyme Q10 can also be low in people with cancer and many metabolic problems.

A recent Belgian study of fifty-eight chronic fatigue patients reported that 45% had very low levels of coenzyme Q_{10} in the blood. Chronic fatigue patients with very low coenzyme Q_{10} levels also had more problems with memory and concentration as compared to chronic fatigue patients with normal of coenzyme Q_{10} in the blood. Other studies have shown that supplementation with 100 milligrams or more daily of coenzyme Q_{10} can significantly increase energy in chronic fatigued elders (Maes 2009).

Carnitine is also often low in chronically fatigue patients as well as in heart failure and cancer patients. Carnitine is a key amino acid found in meat. Carnitine helps transport fats into the mitochondria to be burned as energy. (The mitochondria are cell organelles that are involved in most of the cells energy producing and detoxifying reactions.) A recent Italian study of ninety-six patients over age 70 years reported that supplementation with 2 grams of acetyl-L-carnitine twice daily produced significant improvements in both physical and mental fatigue as compared to patients given placebo (Malaguarmera 2008). Both coenzyme Q_{10} and carnitine are available in drugstores and health food stores without a prescription.

The author urges all chronic fatigue patients to get a good diet with a good protein source three or more times per day (lean meat, fish, eggs, skim milk, cheese) and at least five servings a day of wide range of fruits and vegetables. Chronic fatigue patients should eat frequent small meals, as both skipping meals and eating huge meals can reduce energy levels and result in poorer blood sugar control (Timlin 2007). Foods with high levels of sugar and corn syrup and refined flour (white bread, white rice) should be avoided. Chronic fatigue patients should also take some balanced supplements, which include omega-3 fats, B complex vitamins, magnesium, zinc, coenzyme Q_{10}, and L-carnitine or acetyl-L-carnitine. Many chronic fatigue patients have gradually improved after improving their diet and taking a broad range of food supplements.

A multifaceted approach to treating chronic fatigue with both good nutrition and medication may be needed to completely resolve fatigue. Patients were given a comprehensive nutritional supplementation program including high doses of magnesium, B vitamins, melatonin, and probiotics. Patients were also given other drugs as needed such as antifungal drugs, thyroid hormone, estrogen, testosterone, cortisone, fludrocortisones, and SSRI antidepressants such as Zoloft and Paxil. After three months' treatment, thirty of thirty-two patients reported greatly reduced fatigue (Teitelbaum 2001).

Thyroid Problems and Chronic Fatigue

Thyroid problems are common in elders and can often cause chronic fatigue. In the 65-plus age bracket, about 2-3% of women and 1-2% of men have deficiencies in thyroid hormone (hypothyroidism) (Hueston 2001). Many of these thyroid hormone patients are undiagnosed and untreated. Hypothyroidism can cause many health problems including chronic fatigue, weakness, weight gain, dry skin, hair loss, intolerance to cold, constipation, depression, memory loss, and reduced resistance to infection. The author has seen dozens of thyroid-hormone-deficient chronic fatigue elders improve dramatically when given thyroid hormone.

In the author's opinion, all chronic fatigue patients should receive a complete thyroid panel including testing for TSH (thyroid stimulating hormone) and the thyroid hormones T_3 and T_4.

Sleep Problems Commonly Cause Chronic Fatigue in Seniors

Insomnia is a very common problem that affects about 50% of elders (Neubauer 1999). Diet and exercise can both play a critical role in promoting better sleep.

Eating a well-balanced diet and including a small snack before bedtime can often improve elder sleep (Mayo 2009). Alcohol and caffeine taken late can also disrupt sleep (Mayo 2009). The minerals calcium and magnesium play a major role in calming the body down and promoting sleep; however, these minerals are often low in elders. It is recommended that elders with insomnia problems consume at least 1,000 milligrams of calcium and 500 milligrams of magnesium daily (Holistic Online 2009). Some studies have found that tryptophan, an amino acid found in milk, meats, and fish, has been useful in promoting sleep in elders with insomnia. Probiotic bacteria may also promote better sleep. A study of twenty-nine Japanese adults aged 60 to 81 years reported that consuming yogurt with active cultures of *Lactobacillus helviticus* was associated with significantly better sleep and significantly less insomnia (Yamamura 2009). Milk and yogurt are often recommended as bedtime snacks to promote sleep since they contain high levels of both calcium and tryptophan and yogurt also has probiotic bacteria.

Melatonin is a hormone that plays a key role in the sleep/wake cycle (also called "circadian rhythm"). Analysis of five published studies has found that taking from 1 to 5 milligrams of melatonin at bedtime can significantly reduce insomnia in a majority of adults over age 66 years (Buscemi 2005). Reported side effects of melatonin were very rare and included a few cases of nausea and drowsiness. Some small studies have reported that taking 100 to 600 milligrams of supplemental 5-hydroxytryptophan is associated with less insomnia (Birdsall 1998).

Getting enough physical exercise is also important for promoting good sleep, although exercise should not be done within one hour of bedtime or that may make a person too stimulated to sleep. A study of forty-three older adults found that moderate exercise (walking or low-impact aerobics) for thirty minutes times per week resulted in significantly better sleep and significantly less insomnia (King 1997).

Many elders with chronic fatigue syndrome have undiagnosed or diagnosed sleep apnea.

Sleep apnea, or the frequent stopping of breathing, is very common in seniors. Several estimates report that from 37 to 62% of adults over age 60 years have at least mild sleep apnea, with perhaps about half of these patients having moderate to severe sleep apnea (Norman 2008).

Patients with sleep apnea stop breathing many times in each night. Such periods of breathlessness can last thirty to sixty seconds and can occur hundreds of times per night. This makes sleep very inefficient as the person must partially "wake up" every time apnea occurs in order to resume breathing. Sleep apnea patients often snore and cause their bed partner to lose sleep. During sleep apnea periods, blood pressure often goes up and blood oxygen levels go down.

Sleep apnea increases the risk of high blood pressure, heart attacks, heart failure, strokes, diabetes, obesity, chronic fatigue, decline in mental function, mental depression, driving accidents, and male erectile dysfunction (Hirschkowitz 2008; Karkoulias 2007). Many sleep apnea patients get so tired that they fall asleep while driving or working. Auto accident rates in sleep apnea patients are two to three times that of healthy controls (Barbe 2007).

LUKE CURTIS, MD

Persons most at risk for apnea includes males and large persons with a body mass index (BMI) of more than 30 (see chapter 3 for information about BMI) or a neck circumference of more than 17 inches (Flemons 2002). Smoking or exposure to pesticides and solvents also increases risk of sleep apnea (Al Lawati 2009; Viaene 2009). However, the author has seen sleep apnea in many people who are at "low risk" for sleep apnea, such as slender nonsmoking older women.

He encourages any patient of any age who has prolonged and unexplained chronic fatigue to consult a physician about getting a sleep study. Sleep apnea may be easily diagnosed with the use of overnight sleep testing (polysomnography). This can be performed at a hospital or sleep study center. A sleep study at the hospital is fairly expensive and may cost several thousand dollars. If your insurance does not cover sleep testing, you can ask your physician if a less expensive sleep apnea study can be performed at home. A patient sleeps at home bed while attached to a CPAP machine and oxygen monitor. Such a home sleep test costs several hundred dollars instead of several thousand dollars. The author has performed this home sleep apnea testing successfully for many patients.

Mild sleep apnea can also often be treated with oral appliances used to hold the mouth open during sleep and/or surgery in the mouth and throat (Almedia 2009). For overweight patients, losing weight through diet and exercise can also help reduce the severity of sleep apnea (Hirschkowitz 2008). However, most moderate to severe cases of sleep apnea are usually treated with a machine called a CPAP (continuous positive air pressure breathing machine). A CPAP is a machine that provides air pressure through a tube into a mask that fits over the patient's face. Be sure to clean the CPAP mask and tubing regularly.

The use of continuous positive air pressure (CPAP) pumps and masks has been associated with many improvements in the quality of life including lower blood pressure, reduced risk of heart attacks and strokes, and few driving accidents (Lieberman 2009; Barbe 2007; Karkoulias 2007). The author has seen many older patients improve dramatically after being placed on CPAP. Several patients who were unable to drive or walk a mile were able to resume driving and taking long walks following CPAP treatment.

He remembers one patient in particular who was helped with CPAP treatment. When he first saw her, she was a 64 year old who slept fourteen to sixteen hours per day and was always tired. She had been to forty physicians including several psychiatrists with little relief. She was of moderate weight, a nonsmoker, and her diet and nutrition program seemed to be good. He then suggested she get a sleep study. Her sleep study diagnosed moderate to severe sleep apnea, and she was placed on CPAP treatment. Following CPAP treatment, she recovered in a few months. She resumed working full-time and started jogging, swimming, bicycling, and lifting weights regularly. She then found and married an active man. At age of 70 years, she ran a 26.2 mile marathon in under 4.5 hours!

Despite the obvious advantages of the use of CPAP in treating sleep apnea, many sleep apnea patients refuse to use a CPAP due to problems with masks. The two biggest hurdles to CPAP use are problems in fitting the mask and concerns that the CPAP machine and mask will annoy the sleep partner.

More than one hundred CPAP masks are now commercially available. The author suggests that CPAP patients dissatisfied with their masks try on several different types of CPAP masks to see if these would fit their face better. If you are having trouble getting a CPAP mask fitted to your face, be sure to contact your sleep physicians, sleep study center, or medical supply company for advice on fitting a CPAP mask.

Some patients are afraid to use CPAP masks for fear of what their sleep partner might think. However, they should be reassured that the quality of life also significantly improves for the sleep partner treated with CPAP. Most CPAP machines are quiet (much more quiet than the snoring!) and do not interfere with sleep of the bed partner. Most notably, studies report that the average sleep partner gets significantly more sleep and significantly more sex when the partner is treated with CPAP! (Parish 2003; Karkoulias 2007; Siccoli 2008; Zias 2009). The CPAP mask can be quickly removed to begin sexual activity.

Chemical Exposures, Mold and Chronic Infections Are Also Common Cause of Chronic Fatigue in Elders

Many studies have reported that low-level exposures to such chemicals as pesticides, solvents, carbon monoxide, lead, and mercury can cause chronic fatigue (Pall 2009). If possible, try to avoid pesticide spraying in your home or apartment. Indoor insects can usually be controlled by the use of less toxic means such cleanliness and use of traps that contain flypaper or small amounts of pesticides. To avoid carbon monoxide poisoning inside the home, do not burn wood or charcoal indoors and make sure your heating system is checked every year for possible carbon monoxide emissions.

Heavy mold exposure can also cause severe fatigue. One study reported a group of seventy-nine chronically fatigued patients who were heavily exposed to indoor molds. Of these seventy-nine patients, 51% had a deficiency of growth hormone, while 81% had a deficiency of thyroid hormone (Dennis 2009). A lack of growth hormone and/or thyroid hormone can cause chronic fatigue. It is hypothesized that heavy mold exposure can damage the pituitary gland. The pituitary gland is located just below the brain and is responsible for controlling production of many hormones. Complete or substantial resolution of fatigue was noted in 93% of these patients who were given antifungal medication, antifungal nasal sprays, replacement growth hormone and thyroid hormone, and reduction of their indoor mold exposure (Dennis 2009).

The best way to control indoor mold growth is to prevent water flooding or buildup on building and household materials. To avoid indoor mold problems, make sure that all problems with flooding and wet carpets, walls, floors, and ceilings are corrected within 24 hours.

Many infections can cause chronic fatigue, such as mononucleosis and Lyme disease. Lyme disease is caused by a bacteria called *Borrelia burgdorferi* and spread by the deer tick (*Lxodes scapularis*). Lyme disease causes rashes, low-grade fevers, severe fatigue and can damage the heart and nervous system (Bratton 2005). The author has seen dozens of chronically fatigued Lyme disease patients improve dramatically when given antibiotics to cure their Lyme disease.

Treating Chronic *Candida* (Yeast) Infections Can Cure Chronic Fatigue

Some physicians report that dietary and medication treatment for chronic *Candida* infections are often helpful in improving energy levels. *Candida* are molds (yeasts) that live in the human intestines, but oftentimes can become overgrown (Crook 1986). *Candida* overgrowth is especially common in people who eat large amounts of sugar, who have undergone many antibiotic treatments or who have taken steroid medication like prednisone. A number of published studies have reported that *Candida* overgrowth can produce significant quantities of beverage alcohol (ethanol), the toxic chemical acetaldehyde, and many allergy-causing proteins (Crook 1986).

A *Candida* diet emphasizes vegetables and protein sources like meat, fish, and meats. Refined sugar, corn syrup, alcohol, fruit juices, and yeast containing foods like breads are avoided on a *Candida* diet. Oftentimes, the patient is also prescribed

LUKE CURTIS, MD

antifungal drugs like Diflucan (fluconazole) and also given antifungal supplements and foods such as caprylic acid and garlic to reduce Candida growth. Several excellent books about following a diet to reduce Candida growth in gut have been written by William Crook, MD (*The Yeast Connection*, 1986) and Doug Kaufmann, MS (*The Fungus Link*, volumes 1, 2, and 3).

Published data on the effects of Candida treatment and resolution of chronic fatigue are rather sparse. Carol Jessop, MD, treated 900 of her chronic fatigue patients with the antifungal drug ketoconazole (Nizoral), along with careful diet, which eliminates refined sugar, yeast, alcohol and fruit juices. After three to twelve months of treatment with ketoconazole and an antifungal diet, 529 (59%) patients regained their former health, another 232 (26%) patients showed significant health improvement, and 136 patients (15%) stayed the same or got worse (Jessop 1989). Many of these patients showed resolution of chronic health problems such as vaginal yeast infections, skin rashes, irritable bowel syndrome, depression, and problems with concentration and memory. Much more research on the treatment of chronic Candida problems is needed.

Mild exercise such as walking, slow bicycling, or a moderated pace exercise class is often useful in reducing chronic fatigue in elders (Wick 2007). Severe depression can cause or worsen chronic fatigue. Please see chapter 11 for ideas about combating depression with good nutrition and exercise.

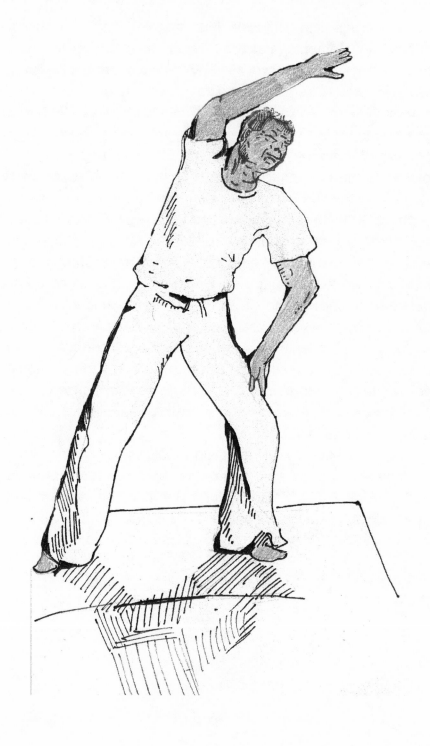

CHAPTER 16

NUTRITION TO TREAT JOINT PROBLEMS

M any elders are bothered by chronic joint problems that cause stiffness, limit their mobility, interfere with work and recreation activities, limit strength, and often cause pain. Oftentimes pain is accompanied by sleep problems. Research exists that arthritis can greatly worsen sleep problems like insomnia, and sleep problems can also worsen arthritis (Smith 2009).

Joint problems have many possible causes, but the most common causes are osteoarthritis, rheumatoid arthritis, mechanical injuries to joints, fibromyalgia, or bone loss (osteoporosis). Chapter 4 has discussed nutritional and exercise treatments for bone loss, while chapter 15 discussed nutritional treatments for fibromyalgia. Cancer can also cause pain/stiffness with bones and joints, so any patient with recent onset of joint or bone pain should consult a physician to rule out cancer. Infections, exposure to toxic chemicals (including mycotoxins from molds), and many different autoimmune diseases such as Sjogren's syndrome, Ankylosing spondylitis, lupus, sarcoidosis can also cause joint problems.

Osteo and Rheumatoid Arthritis
Very Common in Elders

Osteoarthritis is most common chronic joint problem, with 70-90% of adults over age 75 years having at least one affected joint (Hinton 2002). Osteoarthritis involves cartilage degeneration and bone rubbing and is often related to injury or repetitive motion trauma. Osteoarthritis is especially common in knees, hips, feet, shoulders, hands, and distal (outer) joints on each finger. Oftentimes one or more joints are involved in an asymmetric manner (i.e., left side more affected than right or vice versa).

Osteoarthritis is more common among overweight individuals, among inactive persons, or among persons with histories of severe joint injuries (Hinton 2002). A number of studies have reported the pain and stiffness of arthritis is often greatly reduced when a patient loses weight. Please see chapter 3 for more information on weight and health.

Rheumatoid arthritis is also fairly common with about 0.5% of adult men and 1.0% of adult women having rheumatoid arthritis (Klippel 1997). Rheumatoid arthritis involves immunological processes that cause swelling of the synovial fluid located between the joints. Rheumatoid arthritis is especially common in feet, ankles, knees, hands, and proximal (inner) joints on each finger. Morning stiffness of an hour or more duration is common with rheumatoid arthritis. Other features can often develop with rheumatoid arthritis including formation of nodules on skin or lung, subtle neurological changes, anemia, and swelling of the pericardial sac around the heart (Klippel 1997).

Dietary and Exercise Treatments for Arthritis

A number of nutritional treatments exist to treat arthritis. The most commonly used arthritis supplements are chondroitin sulfate and glucosamine. Glucosamine sulfate and chondroitin

LUKE CURTIS, MD

sulfate compounds are found in healthy joint tissue and often become depleted in osteoarthritis patients. Glucosamine and chrondroitin can be manufactured by humans from other dietary components, but research has indicated that older people manufacture significantly less of these compounds than younger people (Richy 2003). Many studies have reported that glucosamine/chrondroitin supplements can restore normal levels of chrondroitin and glucosamine to the joints and significantly reduce pain, stiffness, and swelling of arthritic joints. A review of fifteen double-blind studies of 1,775 middle-aged or elder patients with knee osteoarthritis found that use of either glucosamine or chondroitin sulfate significantly reduced patient reported with knee pain and stiffness as compared to placebo (these results are very statistically significant) (Richy 2003). In addition, seven studies of 755 patients found significantly less joint narrowing in patients receiving glucosamine as compared to placebo ($p<0.001$). Doses in these studies were 1,500 milligram/day for glucosamine and 800 to 2,000 milligram/day for chrondroitin.

Few side effects have been reported with the use of chrondroitin and glucosamine supplementation. The levels of adverse effects side effects in these studies was only 80% the level found in placebo patients (Richy 2003). While glucosamine and chrondroitin are a safe and effective way of treating osteoarthritis, they have to be taken at least daily over a period of several months to get any significant benefit. Chondroitin sulfate and glucosamine must also be taken together for maximum benefit.

A number of studies have reported that consumption of omega-3 fats are associated with significantly improved joint pain and stiffness for both osteo and rheumatoid arthritis patients. Some of these studies have reported that osteo arthritis patients who take omega-3 fats are often able to reduce their consumption of pain killers such as aspirin or ibuprofen. Other studies have reported that supplements of antioxidant vitamins (vitamins A, C, E) or high consumption of fruits and vegetables are associated with significant levels of oxidative stress in the joints and may reduce joint pain and stiffness. Other studies have reported that supplements containing B complex vitamins, vitamin D, magnesium, and zinc may be helpful in reducing arthritis symptoms (Efthomiou 2009). One double-blind study reported that rheumatoid arthritis patients who consumed capsules containing the probiotic bacteria *Lactobacillus rhamnosus* for one year had modest improvements in pain and stiffness as compared to rheumatoid patients given placebo (Hatakka 2003).

S-adenosylmethionine (SAMe) is a compound produced in the liver from the amino acid methionine. Numerous studies have reported that daily supplementation with high doses of SAMe are associated with significant pain reductions in a majority of osteoarthritis patients (Gregory 2008). Some of these studies have reported that the reduction in pain with SAMe is about equal to that produced by taking prescription painkilling drugs like Celebrex (Najm 2004). SAMe is fairly expensive supplement, costing about $30 to $60 per month at a dose of 1,200 milligrams per day. Be sure to shop around for the best prices on SAMe.

A number of herbal supplements show some promise in relieving arthritis symptoms. Such herbs or herbal extracts include cat's claw (*Uncaria tomentosa*), turmeric (*Curcuma longa*), ginger (*Zingiber officinale*), and dandelion (*Taraxacum officinale*). Most of these herbs are helpful by reducing inflation in the joints (Efthomiou 2009).

Other recent research studies have found that the use of pulsed electromagnetic field therapy (PEMF) can also improve arthritis symptoms. Such devices sometimes go by the name of TENS (transcutaneous electrical nerve stimulation). Some, but not all, studies have also reported that acupuncture can also be helpful in reducing pain and inflammation in osteo and rheumatoid arthritis (Efthomiou 2009).

LUKE CURTIS, MD

Moderate exercise is often very useful for many patients with joint problems. Analysis of thirty-two studies involving 3,719 knee osteoarthritis patients reported that the average participant in exercise programs had significant and major reductions in knee pain and stiffness and significantly better overall knee function than those patients not given exercise treatment (Fransen 2008). Water-based exercise problems are often helpful in reducing pain and stiffness in arthritis patients (Rahmann 2009). Many hospitals, rehabilitation clinics, and fitness centers offer land—or water-based exercise classes specifically for folks with joint problems.

It is also vital that patients with joint problems wear comfortable, well-fitted shoes with adequate support. Many shoe stores specialize in selling shoes specifically made for walking and jogging. Many of these shoe stores are staffed by avid walkers or joggers who are expert in finding and fitting the correct shoes for elders. It's oftentimes well worth the investment to spend a bit more money on shoes that are well fitted and offer ample support. Many arthritic patients will also benefit from having orthotic supports in their shoes (Hinman 2009).

Not smoking or quitting is also critical for maintaining joint health. Several studies had reported that tobacco smokers have increase loss of joint cartilage and much slower healing of bone fractures and joint injuries as compared to nonsmokers (Davies-Tuck 2009; Castillo 2005). As stated in chapter 8, quitting smoking is very beneficial to health in many ways even if one has been smoking for decades (Taylor 2002). Many elders have quit smoking with the help of nicotine patches or stop-smoking programs.

Other such environmental exposures can increase risk of rheumatoid arthritis including home and occupational exposure to occupational exposure to silica (sand), pesticides, building moisture damage/mold growth, and hairdresser chemicals (Khuder 2002; Stolt 2005; Luosujarvi 2003). Moderate to severe joint pain/stiffness was found in 71% of a group of forty-eight patients heavily exposed to indoor molds (Lieberman 2003).

Avoiding foods a patient is allergic to can also reduce risk of rheumatoid arthritis, although data is rather sparse. A study of one hundred rheumatic arthritis patients found that about one-third had their symptoms greatly reduced or eliminated for a period of years by eliminating foods they were allergic to (Darlington 1991).

The final three chapters of the book will give specific suggestions to improve the diet and provide proper supplements for elders. These three chapters will also attempt to summarize some of the information of health benefits of proper diet given in earlier chapters.

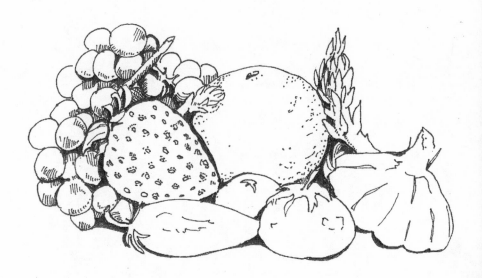

CHAPTER 17

NEAR-IDEAL DIETS: MENU GUIDELINES AND OTHER IDEAS TO IMPROVE ELDER NUTRIENT INTAKES

The previous chapters have discussed the extent and reasons for elder malnutrition and the specific health problems that may be avoided or mitigated by the use of good nutrition. This chapter will give nutritional ideas for seniors and tips on improving their nutritional intake to meet the unique nutritional needs of their age group. Elders with food allergies, religious proscriptions, or specific problems like diabetes may need to make revisions on these dietary suggestions. For specific ideas about what to eat during the day, please see chapter 19 which provides additional menu suggestions.

In general, seniors should try to eat a well-balanced diet consisting of a good protein source (meat, fish, eggs, milk, cheese, or legumes like soybeans) at every meal at least three times daily, at least two daily servings of dairy products and five or more servings of wide variety of fruits and vegetables including sea vegetable like kelp. Fatty fish should be eaten at least twice a week for omega-3 fats. Moderate amounts of whole grains such as whole wheat bread, whole grain cereals, brown rice, and nuts and seeds should also be eaten. Seniors should also consume at least 6 cups a day of water in the form of water, milk, juice, soups, coffee, tea, etc. More fluids should be consumed in the hot weather. The use of sugary foods, refined grain products like white rice and white bread, and alcohol should be limited. To prevent heart disease, stroke, and Alzheimer's, the amounts of saturated fat and trans fats should be limited. For elders with irritable bowel, constipation, or diverticulitis, high fiber foods like oat bran, whole grains, flaxseed, beans, and prunes should be consumed daily along with sufficient amounts of liquid.

Be Sure to Drink at Least Six to Eight Eight-Ounce Glasses of Fluids Daily

Drinking a sufficient liquids is critical for elders, as they oftentimes become dehydrated. Elders need at least six to eight 8-ounce (230 milliliter) glasses of liquids per day and more in hot weather. Many seniors do not drink enough liquids (persons with kidney problems or water retention may have to limit their liquid consumption upon medical advice). Some seniors find drinking water to be boring. However, not all of the liquid consumption has to be in the form of water. In addition to plain water, elders can use flavored water, milk, juice, soup, coffee, tea, and sugar-free colas to obtain their water requirement. Elders often drink more liquids when given a variety of different liquids during the day.

Most elders can tolerate moderate amounts of caffeinated beverages like regular coffee and tea. Some seniors experience problems like trouble sleeping, jitteriness, and fast heartbeat after drinking caffeinated beverages and may have to avoid all caffeine-containing drinks (Smith 2002).

In hot weather, profuse sweating causes loss of many salts or "electrolytes" such as sodium and potassium. Good fluids to drink during hot weather include tomato juice or V-8-type juice, tomato or vegetable soup, or skim milk (all of these foods are rich in both sodium and potassium). Orange and grapefruit juices are rich in potassium but not in sodium. Electrolyte drinks like Gatorade also contain a fair amount of sodium and potassium, but on the negative side, they also often contain lots of refined sugar.

Be Sure to Get Five to Ten Servings of Wide Range of Fruits and Vegetables Daily!

As noted in many chapters in this book, consuming five or ten daily servings (a serving consisted of at least one-half cup) of a wide range of fresh fruits and vegetables are critical for maintaining health and preventing many health problems. Yet only about one-third of elders consume five or more servings of produce a day. Vegetables and fruits are rich in water, fiber, minerals, and vitamins. Fruits and vegetables also continue a wide variety of plant-synthesized chemicals called "phytochemicals", which fight heart disease, strokes, vision problems, cancer, infection, allergy, and many other health problems.

At least one serving daily of dark green or yellow vegetables like broccoli, carrots, pumpkin, sweet potatoes, parsley, spinach, leaf lettuce, mustard greens, etc., should be eaten for their rich supply of beta-carotene (a form of vitamin A). Every day, at least one serving of a vitamin C-rich fruit or vegetable such as citrus fruits (oranges, grapefruits, tangerines, etc.); melons; kiwi; strawberries; broccoli; tomatoes; peppers; or potatoes should also be eaten. Red/purple grapes and berries (especially blueberries) are very rich in phytochemicals and should be eaten regularly. Allium family vegetables (onions, garlic, chives) and Cruciferous family vegetables (broccoli, cabbage) should be eaten at least every other day for their strong anticancer properties.

Some people complain that eating vegetables are boring. However, vegetables can be prepared in a number of interesting ways including being eaten raw, being made into salads, or being steamed, baked or stir-fried or added to soups, chili, or meat or fish dishes. Inexpensive steamers are sold at most grocery stores. These steamers allow many vegetables like broccoli and green beans to be steam prepared in only three to six minutes. White and sweet potatoes can easily be prepared by microwaving them for several minutes. Chili can be prepared with many nutritious vegetables such as tomatoes, peppers, onions, carrots, and parsley/cilantro.

Don't neglect salads. A large number of vegetables are great in green salads such as leaf lettuce, spinach, arugula, radish, watercress, artichoke, broccoli, parsley, carrots, cucumber, tomatoes, peppers, onions, and many other vegetables. *Use your imagination when mixing salads!* Sprouted seeds of radish, alfalfa, broccoli, and onion are nutritional powerhouses that are also great in green salads. The author loves the strong and delicious taste of onion sprouts when mixed with other blander salad vegetables. Many supermarkets offer many interesting prepared salad mixes. Try to eat green salads prepared with salad dressings prepared with flax, soybean, walnut, or canola oil in order to get a good blend of both omega-3 and omega-6 fatty acids. Eating coleslaw (cabbage) and broccoli slaw are good ways to get more of the important cruciferous vegetables.

If any of your family or friends joke that vegetables are "rabbit food", please remind them that vegetables are also "gorilla food". Gorillas are very strong primates that eat huge amounts of vegetables.

Melons like watermelon, cantaloupe, and honeydew are very refreshing, especially in hot weather. Melons can be eaten plain or combined with other fruits, yogurt, or cottage cheese. Grapes, blueberries, and other berries are great on cereals, in whole grain breads and muffins, in fruit, vegetable, and meat dishes, or just eaten plain by the hand. Apples, pears, oranges, and bananas are nutritious fruits that are easy to carry and to eat with your hands. Many hikers and bicyclists snack on fruits during long walks/rides.

Fruits and vegetables also make good smoothies in the blender. A favorite smoothie of the author consists of blending 1 small banana, 1 small bunch of grapes or 4 ounces of blueberries, 1 carrot, and 5 sprigs of parsley in a blender with a half cup of water. Most supermarkets also sell commercial fruit and vegetable juices like V-8. However, smoothies are more nutritious than juices since smoothies still contain the fiber from fruits and vegetables.

Saving Money on Fruits and Vegetables

Some elders express concerns about the availability and cost of fruits and vegetables. Elders who live in some rural areas and inner-city neighborhoods may have limited selection of fruits and vegetables at the nearest store. Fruits and vegetables may also be fairly expensive, especially if out of season. How can one obtain a wide variety of fresh fruits and vegetables at reasonable prices? Customers should check local stores for sales on fruits and vegetables. Elders are often enthusiastic newspaper readers and clippers. Shoppers can save 20-30% on their total food bills by using newspaper coupons. Oftentimes, smaller fruit/vegetable stands/stores, Hispanic markets, or large warehouse-style stores like ALDI offer produce at considerably cheaper prices than traditional supermarkets. Considerable savings can sometimes be had by buying produce such as potatoes, carrots, onions, apples, oranges, and grapefruit in large bags of 3 to 10 pounds. Be sure to store fruits and vegetables promptly in the refrigerator and throw out any produce that becomes rotten or moldy.

Many towns have weekly farmers markets that offer a wide range of organic fruits and vegetables at reasonable prices. Some areas also have subscription farming in which for a flat fee customers receive a percentage of fresh organic fruits and vegetables grown on a farm. In years of abundant harvests, subscription farming is often far cheaper than buying produce at the supermarket. Many communities have cooperative groceries that offer much cheaper food prices to members in exchange for working at the co-op several hours per week.

Frozen fruits and vegetables are almost as nutritious as their fresh counterparts and are often much cheaper, especially for out-of-season produce. For example, in December 2009 in Chicago, fresh blueberries from Chile cost about $10 a pound while frozen blueberries from Michigan or Quebec cost only $3 per pound.

Home Gardens Can Produce Delicious Fruits and Vegetables and Save Money

Growing your own fruits and vegetables is another way to save money on produce. This writer obtained his love of gardening almost entirely from working with his grandparents and other older adults who were garden experts. A wide variety of fruits and vegetables can be grown in most parts of the USA as long as the garden receives at least a half-day of sun. The soil can be fertilized and conditioned by adding free materials such as composted leaves, grass clippings, and kitchen scraps like eggshells and fruit peels.

Many plants like lettuce, corn, parsley, and green beans can be easily grown from seeds. Keep the ground wet until seedlings are well established. Other plants like tomatoes, peppers, melons, and broccoli and are best placed in the garden as seedlings to give them a head start on growth. Started plants can be purchased at garden centers or grown inside in a sunny window in late winter.

Leafy vegetables such as lettuce, parsley, dandelions, mustard greens are both easy to grow and very nutritious. Two or three crops of lettuce can be grown each year. The author is a

LUKE CURTIS, MD

parsley fanatic who plants and harvests several hundred parsley plants each year to give away and for his own use.

Another especially nutritious group of plants are the cruciferous vegetables, which include broccoli, brussels sprouts, cauliflower, kale, cabbage, bok choy, and radish. The cruciferous vegetables are named for their cross-shaped flowers and are easy to grow in home gardens. Cruciferous vegetables are very rich in vitamins and minerals. Cruciferous vegetables also contain several phytochemicals that have strong anticancer properties (please see chapter 9 for information about cruciferous vegetables and their anticancer properties). Broccoli is an especially nutritious vegetable that has a very long growing season of five to six months. Broccoli plants can be placed in the ground in April and the large main flower stems harvested in June or early July. Keep the broccoli plants well watered and they will continue producing delicious smaller side shoots of broccoli flowers until heavy frost finally kills the plants in November or December.

In sunny locations, tomatoes and cucumbers often yield heavily in a small area. Delicious melons such as watermelon, honeydew, cantaloupe, and pumpkin can be easily grown in home gardens that offer the large space (10 to 30 feet) that these melons require. Sweet corn is also delicious crop that is easy to grow but requires a lot of space. White and sweet potatoes can be easily grown by planting small potato fragments or "eyes". Onions can be easily grown by planted small onions or "sets". Carrots are easy to grow but require a loose soil full of sand and organic matter in order to reach large size.

Dwarf versions of fruit trees such apples, pears, cherries, and peaches are very convenient. Small versions of oranges and grapefruit are also great for frost free areas. Dwarf fruit trees take up little space, start bearing after a few years, and are short enough to be harvested while standing on the ground or on a short ladder. Two different varieties of some fruit trees may have to be planted for cross-pollination. After they are established for five to ten years, the yields from dwarf or semidwarf fruit trees can be surprisingly heavy. The author's grandfather had two semidwarf apple and two semidwarf pear trees in his small parsonage backyard. Each of these semidwarf fruit trees produced several hundred pounds of fruit each fall! Grapes are also fairly easy to grow in home gardens. Purple varieties of grapes have the highest quantities of revasterol and other beneficial phytochemicals.

For apartment dwellers, many towns offer community garden plots available for rent at a small cost. Some vegetables like tomatoes, parsley, and leaf lettuce can also be grown on sunny porches by apartment dwellers. Some city buildings offer opportunities for rooftop gardening. A Chicago organic restaurant called Uncommon Ground grows much of its organic herbs and vegetables on the roof of its building.

In addition to providing excellent organic fruits and vegetables, gardening also provides an excellent opportunity for exercise, giving excess produce to neighbors, and getting vitamin D from sunlight. Some folks may require sunblock for extended sun exposure (more than thirty minutes when the sun is above 30 degrees from the horizon), especially if they are fair skinned or burn easily.

Don't Forget about Eating Delicious Sea Vegetables

Sea vegetables are rich in many phytochemicals and minerals (especially iodine) and should be eaten more often. Sea vegetables make a delicious side dish or can be added to soups, meats, fish, and land vegetables for flavoring. People in many seaside regions such as Japan, coastal China, Polynesia, Hawaii, Alaska, Chile, Ireland, Denmark, and Scotland have regularly eaten sea vegetables for centuries. Kelp (*Alaria esculenta*) can be used as salty seasoning in many soups, vegetables, eggs, fish and meats. Irish moss (*Chondrus crispus*) can be made into a thick pudding. Rockweed (*Fucus pesicylosus*) can be cooked into a delicious crunchy vegetable. Dulse (*Palmaria palmata*) has a nutty flavor that is great eaten by itself or added to potatoes, breads, and soups (Brill 1994). Sea vegetables are readily available in many large supermarkets and Asian food shops.

Get Enough Omega-3 Fats for Good Health

Many chapters of this book have talked about the importance of getting enough omega-3 fatty acids. How can elders get more fish in their diet? The easiest way of getting omega-3 fats in your diet is to eat at least three meals a week containing at least a 3-ounce serving of fatty fish such as salmon, mackerel, anchovies, sardines, and herring. These fatty fish can be prepared in many interesting ways such as baking, broiling, frying, adding to soups, or being eaten cold on whole grain bread or crackers. Using flax oil for cooking or salad dressing or by adding flax seed to cereals and breads are another good way to increase omega-3 consumption in your diet. The use of soybean, canola and evening primrose oils, pumpkin seeds, and walnuts can also add omega-3 fats to your diet. For more information about levels of omega-3 fats in foods, please see omega-3 section in chapter 18.

Most commercially grown meat, milk, and eggs are low in omega-3 fats. Several studies have reported that meat and milk from pastured cattle and buffalo (bison) have higher omega-3 levels than cattle fed standard feedlot diets (Dannenberger 2007). The author knows of one fish-allergic 70-year-old woman who gets her omega-3 from meat and milk from pastured animals. This woman is still working a full-time job, spending time with grandchildren, and maintaining a small farm with dairy goats. Some eggs with higher levels of omega-3 fats are available from hens fed special diets.

Omega-3 from fish oil is available in both liquid form (such as fish oil or cod-liver oil) or in capsules containing fish oil. Fish oil is much less expensive than the capsules if you can stand the fishy taste. Store cod-liver oil and fish oil in the refrigerator to keep it fresh and to reduce the fishy taste. Many stores also sell flavored cod-liver oil to reduce the fishy taste. Many horror stories about the terrible taste of cod-liver oil involved eating old rancid oil that has not been refrigerated. Fresh, refrigerated cod-liver oil should have a fairly mild taste. For maximum health benefits, plan on taking at least one teaspoon (4 milliliters) of cod liver or fish oil or at least four large capsules (1,000 milligrams each) of fish oil daily

It should be noted that fatty fish, fish oil, and cod-liver oil are all very rich in both omega-3 fats and vitamin D, which are two vital nutrients that are deficient in a majority of seniors' diets.

Get a Good Source of Protein at Least Three Times Daily

Eating good protein sources such as meat, fish, milk, cheese, eggs, and legumes such as peanuts and soybeans are essential to maintain good health. Avoid fatty cuts of meat such as sirloin steak, ribs, hot dogs, and regular sausage, since commercial-raised beef and pork fat is largely saturated. Lower fat versions of many meat products such as hamburger, hot dogs, and sausage are now available. Much of the fat from some cuts of meat can be eliminated through cooking, for example much of the fat from hamburgers can be drained away or blotted with a paper or cloth towel. In addition, many soybean-based "meat" products are now available which are rich in protein and low in saturated fats.

Elders should plan on eating 1 to 1.5 grams of protein per kilogram (2.2 pounds) of bodyweight daily. For a table of protein content in common foods, please see the protein section in chapter 18.

Eggs should be eaten regularly by elders. Eggs are a very nutritious food, inexpensive and easy to prepare in many interesting ways. For example, omelets are easy to prepare in a nonstick pan and many nutritious and delicious ingredients like milk, cheese, onions, broccoli, spinach, tomatoes and other herbs, spices, and seasonings can be easily added. Eggs have very high-quality protein that contains all of the essential amino acids in abundance. This high-quality egg protein is especially important for people recovering from infection, surgery, or accidental trauma. Eggs are one of the richest sources of methionine, a sulfur containing amino acid that is helpful to fight infection, rebuild tissue, and detoxify many harmful chemicals. Eggs also contain lutein, a chemical necessary for proper vision and for reducing the risk of age-related macular degeneration.

Eggs are also fairly rich in cholesterol, with about 225 milligrams of cholesterol per whole egg. Eggs also contain about many other nutrients, including lecithin, a fatty substance that helps to lower cholesterol in the blood. In the 1970s and 1980s, many people avoided eating eggs for fear of high blood cholesterol. However, numerous studies have reported that eating up to two eggs daily is not associated with higher blood cholesterol levels or higher rates of heart disease and stroke (Song 2000; Qureshi 2007).

At least two or three servings of dairy products such as milk, yogurt, and cheese should be eaten daily for protein and calcium, unless the person is allergic to milk. Lower fat milk (such as 1% and 2%) and cheese are generally preferable to full-fat versions. Some people are lactose intolerant and cannot digest the lactose (sugar) in milk. These persons can usually tolerate milk very well if they take digestive enzymes containing lactose (such as Lactaid).

Elders allergic to cow's milk should consider drinking delicious goat's milk. Many people who are allergic to cow's milk can tolerate goat's milk (Restani 1999). Goat's milk is rich in protein and calcium and has a richer flavor than cow's milk, although it is lower than folate content than cow's milk.

For better sleep and digestion, either milk products with probiotic bacteria or probiotic bacteria capsules should be consumed at least once a week. Most yogurts also contain live probiotic bacteria such as *Lactobacillus* and *Bifidobacterium*, which are helpful for digestion and immunity. To save money, yogurt-making machines are available, which produce yogurt cheaply from store-bought milk. If a person cannot tolerate dairy products at all, they should take at least 1,000 milligrams a day of a calcium supplement.

Nuts, Seeds, and Whole Grains Provide Important Nutrients

Nuts and seeds are rich in protein, unsaturated fats, fiber, and many vitamins and minerals. Nuts are concentrated sources of nutrition that are delicious and easy to store and carry. Nuts and seeds can be added to many meat, fish, egg, and vegetable dishes and added to whole grain cereals, breads, and fruit dishes. The high protein and calorie content of nuts and seeds makes them ideal for elders who need to maintain or gain weight. On the other hand, eating small amounts of nuts may be helpful in preventing weight gain in heavy elders. Several published studies of adults have reported that eating 1 to 3 ounces of nuts and nut butters daily over a three to six months results in little weight change. Adults who ate small amounts of nuts tended to reduce their intake of less healthy foods containing large amount of sugar and refined grain products like white bread. In addition, energy levels and rates of calorie burning were generally increased in the adults given nuts in their diet (Mattes 2007). As noted in chapter 8, walnuts are especially helpful in lowering levels of LDL or bad cholesterol.

LUKE CURTIS, MD

Many large supermarkets and health food stores have a wide range of nuts and nut butters for sale including peanuts, soybeans, almonds, pecans, cashews, walnuts, filberts, brazil nuts, hazelnuts, as well as pumpkin, sunflower, hemp, and sesame seeds. Avoid moldy nuts, as many nuts (especially peanuts) are often contaminated with toxic mold (fungi) and mold toxins called mycotoxins. A mold called aflatoxin often grows on stale corn and peanuts. Aflatoxin exposure can increase risk of liver and lung cancer (Wild 2010). To reduce the risk of mold contamination, many people store nuts and nut butters in the refrigerator. Nut butters are very tasty on whole grain breads and on many raw fruits and vegetables.

Breads and cereals should be eaten in moderation by most seniors, unless they are underweight and/or very active and need the calories. Eating too many breads and cereals can crowd out other nutritious foods like fruits, vegetables, meats, fish, cheese, and dairy products. Breads and cereals products should always be whole grain, as much of the nutrients and fiber are removed in processing grain. Use 100% whole wheat bread or whole grain breads, whole grain cereals like oatmeal, popcorn, and brown rice. Be sure to check the labels of breads and cereals as many breads that say they are "wheat" or "whole grain" are mostly white (refined) flour. Whole grain flours can be purchased at most health food stores and used to make delicious bread, muffins, and pancakes. Soybean grits or flour can be added to whole grain cereals or baked goods for more protein, calcium, iron, and other nutrients. Elders with cholesterol problems should regularly eat oatmeal, oat brain, and soy proteins to lower their LDL or bad cholesterol. Grapes, berries, and nuts can also be added to whole grain cereals, pancakes, and breads for added nutrition and flavor.

Be Sure to Eat a High Protein Breakfast Every Day!

It is important to eat breakfast regularly. Skipping breakfast in the elderly has been associated with significantly higher rates of heart disease, poorer blood sugar control in diabetics, lower levels of energy, and significantly higher death rates (Timlin 2007).

Be sure to eat a breakfast containing a good source of protein such as milk, yogurt, cheese, eggs, lean meat, or fish. Breakfast should always include at least one serving of fruits and vegetables. Fruits may be eaten raw, added to cereal, or made into juice. Vegetables can be eaten raw (carrots and tomatoes), added to egg/meat dishes, or make into juice. If cereals, pancakes, or bread are eaten at breakfast, they should always be 100% whole grain. Avoid sugary breakfast items like donuts, pastry, and sugary cereals. Maple and corn syrups are very high in refined sugar and should be avoided. The author has enjoyed preparing and eating pancakes made with whole grain barley or whole millet flour topped off with fresh fruit instead of syrup. Breakfast is also a convenient time to take food supplements.

As noted in chapter 7, another way to improve nutritional intake for seniors with a poor appetite is the use of nutritional drinks like Boost or Ensure. These drinks are available in many flavors and contain balance amounts of water, protein, fats, carbohydrates, vitamins, minerals, and fiber. Some of the new drinks like Peptamen (Nestlé) contain additional important ingredients such as glutamine or omega-3 fatty acids. Some of these drinks contain a fair amount of sugar and may not be appropriate for those with diabetes. Special low-sugar drinks like Glucerna (Nestlé) are available for diabetic persons.

LUKE CURTIS, MD

Avoid Eating Empty Calories from Sugars, Refined Grains, and Trans/Saturated Fats

Foods rich in refined sugar from sugarcane, beets, corn syrup, or honey should be limited by seniors. Sugars contain "empty calories" with few nutrients and can cause wild swings in blood sugar that can be hard on diabetic. Sugar is present in many processed foods and baked goods and is found in especially large amounts in soft drinks. Nondiet forms of cola such as Coke and Pepsi contain about 40 grams of sugar or corn syrup per 16-ounce serving and should be avoided. The author has seen many elders consume four or more cans of sugar containing cola a day, which amounts to 480 or more empty calories. Instead of regular colas, elders should drink water, milk, juice, or moderate quantities of coffee, tea, and sugar-free soft drinks.

Use of margarines, hydrogenated peanut butter (no oil on top), potato chips, donuts, and other products with "hydrogenated" or trans fats should also be avoided. Be sure to buy "natural" peanut butter with oil on top and no hydrogenated oils added. Fried products like french fries and deep-fried fish are rich in trans fatty acids and should be prepared in other ways. For example, delicious baked potatoes can easily be prepared by microwaving them for three to five minutes. Potatoes can be easily boiled or made into mashed potatoes. Be sure to retain the skin of the potatoes for maximum nutrition. Fish can be easily baked or poached instead of deep-fried.

Commercial donuts are an especially bad food since they are loaded with both trans-fats and refined sugars. One large study of adults over age 84 years reported that consuming donuts four or more times per week was associated with significantly higher rates of heart attacks and a significantly higher overall death rate (Fraser 1997). Elders wanting a sweet snack should enjoy eating fruit instead.

Eating healthy should also mean eating delicious. If you fill up on good-sized portions of fruits, vegetables, lean meat, fish, and low-fat dairy products, you will have less appetite for sugary goodies and trans fat-containing products like donuts and potato chips. As noted in chapter 2, many elders love sweets. If you love sweets, try to enjoy the natural sweet goodness of fruits or plain yogurt. Sweet lovers should also consider buying or preparing delicious deserts with no refined sugars such as sugar-free versions of ice cream, pudding, pumpkin pie, and fruit pies. If you must have refined sugar-containing goodies such as cookies and cake, try to limit yourself to small portions.

Dental Implants, Speech and Swallowing Therapy, and Grinding/Pureeing Food Can Improve Nutritional Status

As noted in chapter 2, many seniors have lost many teeth and about 40% of the US population over age 75 years has a complete set of dentures (Douglass 2000). Elders with dentures have significantly lower intakes of nutritious foods such as meat, fruits, and vegetables and have much greater risk of nutritional deficiencies as compared to elders with their original teeth (Quandt 2009; Walls 2004). Several studies have reported that dental implants are often more comfortable and offer significantly better strength and chewing ability than standard dentures. Patients with dental implants are also significantly less likely to be malnourished than patients with standard dentures. Various studies have reported significantly higher intakes of protein, calories, fiber, and many vitamins and minerals in patients with dental implants as compared to patients with standard dentures (De Oliveira 2004; Hutton 2002). The author strongly urges all elders who have lost many or all of their teeth to consult with a dentist about possibly getting some dental implants installed. Nutritional counseling can also significantly increase consumption of meat, fruits, and vegetables to those with artificial teeth (Bradbury 2006).

Elders with missing teeth can also benefit from eating nutritious prepared foods that required less chewing such as ground meats and chopped or pureed fruits and vegetables. Blenders and food processors to grind and pure meats, fruits, and vegetables can be purchased for less than $25.

Social Factors, Eating Assistance, and Swallowing Therapy Can Greatly Improve Seniors' Nutrition

Social supports can also substantially improve elders' nutrition. Joining cooking clubs, dining out clubs, and gardening clubs are also good ways to improve your nutrition, taste new foods and improve your food variety, and meet interesting people as well. Many seniors like to swap favorite recipes, review local restaurants, or exchange knowledge of growing delicious fruits and vegetables. Some seniors like to take turns serving each other meals in one another's homes/apartments.

Eating with pleasant people and in pleasant surroundings also frequently improves dietary intake of seniors. Several studies have reported that seniors consume significantly more food and have a significantly higher intake of protein, vitamins, and minerals when eating in groups rather than alone (Wright 2006). Residents of elder facilities have better food consumption when eating in dining rooms rather than in their bedrooms. Other studies have noted that use of good tableware and china, flowers on the dining table and use of soft music is associated with significantly better nutritional intake and health status in elders (Mathey 2001).

Seniors who live alone can often benefit by having relatives, friends, and neighbors join them for meals at home or in restaurants. In some communities, seniors can get meals from programs like Meals on Wheels or eat many inexpensive meals at churches and other organizations. Many restaurants offer reduced-priced meals during certain times of the week for those over a certain age such as 65, 60, or even 50 years!

As noted in chapter 7 on hospital nutrition, frail seniors have much better nutritional intakes when people help them eat (Mathey 2001). About 15% of all elders have trouble swallowing (Humbert 2008). Seniors with swallowing difficulties may require adding a thickener like corn starch to beverages. Seniors with swallowing problems can often improve dramatically after getting therapy with a speech/swallowing therapist and doing regular speaking and swallowing exercises (Logemann 2007). The author urges all seniors with swallowing problems to contact a speech/ swallowing therapist. He has seen many tube-fed elders who were too weak to eat food normally who then received speech and swallowing therapy for a month or two and were then able to eat again normally by mouth.

As noted in chapter 2, many low-income seniors are not taking advantage of Federal and State food assistance programs like the Supplemental Nutrition Assistance Program (SNAP). Many communities offer services like Meals on Wheels or elder dining programs that offer well-balanced meal on a sliding scale based on seniors' income. Low-income seniors should investigate these food support opportunities in their communities.

Ideally, elders should get most of their nutrients from a well-balanced diet. However, most seniors will also benefit from taking food supplements as well. The next chapter will give suggestions about a nutritional supplementation program to help seniors obtain and maintain ideal health.

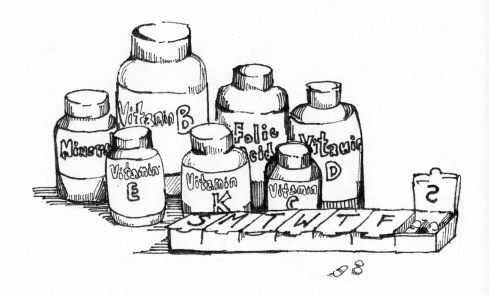

CHAPTER 18

SUPPLEMENT SUGGESTIONS FOR SENIORS: WHY YOU NEED SUPPLEMENTS NOW EVEN IF YOU DID NOT NEED THEM IN MIDDLE AGE

The cornerstone of good nutrition is three or more well-balanced meals daily. Supplements cannot replace a proper diet. Taking food supplements should not be taken an excuse to eat poorly. While a good diet is essential, many researches have indicated that elders will benefit from taking food supplements. As noted in chapter 2, the majority of US seniors simply do not consume enough of many nutrients such as vitamins D, B_{12}, folate, and calcium to maintain optimum health. Even when eating a well-balanced diet, most elders will require some food supplements for vibrant health. The nutritional needs and stresses of seniors require just about all seniors to take some supplements, even though these people may have enjoyed good health in middle age without food supplements.

While many seniors recognize the importance of food supplements, they are often confused as to what supplements to take. Many elders are already consuming food supplements. A survey of 1,825 Massachusetts adults over age 60 years reported that 40% take vitamin/minerals supplements daily (Radimer

2004). However, many seniors taking nutritional supplements do not enjoy their full benefits because they take doses of nutrients that are too low, do not include enough nutrients in their supplementation program, and/or take supplements erratically. This chapter will attempt to give information and guidelines about what are the proper types and doses of food supplements for people to take in their golden years.

Possible Toxic Effects of Food Supplements

Many physicians and medical articles warn against the toxic effects of taking too high a dose of vitamin and mineral supplements. While deficiency of nutrients such as vitamins and minerals is much more common, it is possible to overdose on supplements containing vitamins and minerals. Such vitamin and mineral overdoses are quite rare and are usually confined to a few types of nutrients such as vitamin A and iron. Adults and children have occasionally gotten vitamin A toxicity after consuming 100,000 international units or more per day for months (Merck 2007). As little as 150 milligrams of iron supplements can be toxic to small children as small children have a very limited capacity to handle large amounts of iron as compared to adults (Robotham 1980). Use of weight loss "supplements" containing drugs like ephedra and gamma hydroxyl butyric acid (GHB) have been linked to about five deaths per year in the United States (Saul 2008). Heavy doses of niacin supplements can cause skin flushing (eMed TV 2008). Excessive amounts of some supplements like magnesium and vitamin C can cause diarrhea and/or be used to treat constipation (Natural Cures 2010). Obviously, supplements should be kept away from pets and small children.

It should be noted that using vitamin, mineral, and other supplements are much safer than using either prescription drugs or over-the-counter drugs like aspirin. In the decade of the 2000s, overdoses of conventional vitamin and mineral supplements have

LUKE CURTIS, MD

been estimated to cause about one death per year in the USA, while adverse side effects of prescription and over-the-counter drugs has been estimated at 106,000 deaths per year (Fraser 2005).

Be Sure to Shop Around for Best Supplement Prices

Prices on supplements vary greatly, so be sure to shop local stores, catalogue outfits, and the Internet for best buys on supplements. Oftentimes supplements can be purchased more cheaply in large quantities of 100 to 500 pills or tablets. Oftentimes supplements are cheaper if purchased as combined products such as combination on glucosamine and chondroitin sulfate rather than purchasing each supplement individually. Some products such as cod liver or fish oil are much cheaper purchased as liquid rather than in pill form. Many companies make multivitamin/mineral tablets designed for seniors. Such tablets are often much cheaper than buying supplements for single nutrients. However, many of these multivitamin/mineral tablets are low in some nutrients such as calcium, magnesium, and vitamin C and completely lack other important supplements like omega-3 fats, L-carnitine, and coenzyme Q_{10}. Many elders use a good senior multivitamin/mineral tablet supplemented with separate supplements of calcium, magnesium, vitamin C, omega-3 fats, L-carnitine, and coenzyme Q_{10}.

Liquid supplements and powdered supplements (which can be reconstituted in water, milk, or juice) are available for elders who have trouble swallowing large tablets. Be sure to check labels for nutrient levels when buying supplements. Supplement prices vary greatly, so be sure to shop around for the best prices.

Suggested Supplement Levels for Seniors

The following sections provide recommended levels of supplementation for persons 65 years or older. It is important that all of the essential nutrients be consumed daily, as many nutrients act in concert with other nutrients and can't function when one nutrient is missing. Persons with specific medical conditions like kidney failure or taking specific drugs made need different amounts of these supplements. All of these supplements are available over the counter. A brief description of the function of each nutrient will also be provided as well. Readers wanting fuller information on supplements should consult a comprehensive book on food supplements such as *The Encyclopedia of Nutritional Supplements* by Michael Murray MD (Three Rivers Press, New York City, 1996). Readers may also want to consult a biochemistry textbook to learn more about the structure and function of many nutrients. Seniors with specific health problems can also often benefit by consulting with a good nutritionist or nutrition-minded physician, chiropractor, or nurse. Some nutrition professionals offer blood tests for nutrients that can help to diagnose nutritional deficiencies and provide guidance as to what supplements are needed.

Protein and Protein Supplements

Protein plays a vital role in building and maintaining muscles, bones, blood, organs, and other tissues. Protein is also required to make enzymes that facilitate many chemical reactions in the body. Protein is also required to fight infections and to build many hormones. Proteins are comprised of twenty different amino acids, which include nine "essential amino acids" that must be found in everyone diets. The nine essential amino acids are arginine, isoleucine, leucine, lysine, methionine, phenylalanine, threonine, tryptophan, and valine. Eleven of the amino acids are considered "nonessential" in that the body can make these amino acids if the nine essential amino acids are present in the diet. The eleven nonessential amino acids are alanine, asparagine, aspartate, cysteine, glutamate, glycine, proline, series, tyrosine,

LUKE CURTIS, MD

and histidine. Under conditions of stress like illness or trauma, some "nonessential" amino acids such as glutamine, cysteine, proline, histidine, and tyrosine can become depleted and are considered "conditionally essential" amino acids that must be included in the diet (Wikipedia 2010). Other amino acids like taurine, carnitine, and creatine are also important. For a fuller description of amino acids, please consult a basic biochemistry textbook or Web site such as Wikipedia.

It is generally recommended that seniors consume 1.0 to 1.2 grams of protein per kilogram (2.2 pounds) of body weight daily (Whitney 2008). An elder weighing 70 kilograms or 154 pounds should therefore consume at least 70 grams of protein per day. Some evidence suggests that a higher protein consumption of about 1.5 grams per kilogram per day is useful for elders with muscle loss (sarcopenia) (Kim 2010). Kidney failure patients need to eat a moderate amount of protein amounting to about 1.0 to 1.2 grams of protein daily. Too much protein can be hard on the kidneys, while too little protein can break down tissue (Clements 2006). For patients with normal kidney and liver function, eating too much protein is rarely a problem.

The following table (Whitney 2008) lists protein in common foods. All animal proteins are complete except gelatin. A complete protein means it contains all of the amino acids in proper proportions to sustain life. The protein quality in milk or whey and whole eggs are considered to be nearly perfect proteins for humans.

Plant proteins are generally less complete than animal proteins, although some plant proteins such as soybeans and wheat germ are considered complete. Grains are generally deficient in the amino acids tryptophan and methionine while they contain adequate levels of isoleucine and lysine. Legumes like soybeans, beans, and lentils are deficient in isoleucine and lysine, but generally contain sufficient methionine and tryptophan (Whitney 2008). Eating beans with grains at the same time can provide a complete protein dish.

For the best balance of amino acids, be sure to eat plant proteins with a least a small amount of animal protein. Adding milk to cereal or adding a small amount or meat, fish, eggs, or cheese to bean or pasta dishes can greatly improve the protein quality of the plant sources.

TABLE OF PROTEIN IN COMMON FOODS (From U Healthy, 2010)	
Food	Grams of Protein per Serving
ANIMAL FOODS	
Chicken, boneless, cooked	27
Turkey, roasted, 3 ounces	23
Roast beef or round steak, lean, 3 ounces	24
Ground beef or ground turkey, lean, 3 ounces	23
Pork, lean, roasted, 3 ounces	25
Ham, 3 ounces	23
Tuna, 3 ounces	23
Salmon, 3 ounces	22
Cod, 3 ounces	20
Milk, skim or whole, 8 ounces	8
Yogurt, 8 ounces	8-11
Cheese, hard like cheddar or mozzarella	7-9
Eggs, 1 large	7
PLANT FOODS	
Tofu, ¼ cup	10
Soy grits, ½ cup	15
Peanut butter, ¼ cup	16
Kidney, black or navy beans, cooked, ½ cup	8
Almonds, 1.5 ounce	9
Sunflower seeds, 2 ounces	13
Walnuts, ¼ cup	5
Wheat germ, ¼ cup	8
Whole wheat bread, 1 slice	3
Oatmeal, cooked, 1 cup	6
Brown rice, cooked, 1 cup	5
Pasta, whole wheat, cooked, 1 cup	7

LUKE CURTIS, MD

Protein supplements are useful for elders who have difficulty consuming the recommended 1.0 to 1.5 grams of protein per kilogram per day in their regular diet. Many protein supplements are available in health food stores. Particularly useful is whey protein isolate. Whey protein has an excellent balance of amino acids that are well absorbed in the gut and stimulates protein synthesis in the elderly (Hayes 2008). Several studies have shown that protein supplementation with whey or milk protein can significantly increase muscle mass in seniors in muscle loss (sarcopenia) (Kim 2010). Nutritional drinks like Ensure or Boost are also good ways to increase the daily protein intake.

Amino Acid Supplements

While many protein sources such as milk, meat, fish, eggs, and soybeans contain a "complete" assortment of amino acids, many seniors can benefit from supplementation with one or more of the following six amino acids.

L-Carnitine

L-carnitine is any amino acid that is involved in transporting fats into the mitochondria where they are burned for energy. (The mitochondria are organelles in cells where most of the body's energy-producing reactions occur.) L-carnitine also stimulates a number of enzymes that produce energy for the body. L-carnitine is found in small quantities in the diet in meat and milk. As noted earlier in this book, L-carnitine supplementation can produce significant health benefits to heart patients, patients with macular degeneration, chronically fatigued patients, and men with erectile dysfunction.

No toxic effects of L-carnitine have been reported. The usual recommended level of daily supplementation is 1,000 to 6,000 milligrams a day, divided in two or more doses throughout the day. The author urges all patients with concerns about heart and eye health, chronic fatigue, or erectile dysfunction to consider taking supplemental L-carnitine. Carnitine is a fairly expensive supplement (about 50¢ to $1.50 per 1,000 milligrams), so be sure to shop around health food stores and mail order outlets for the best prices.

L-Taurine

L-taurine is another amino acid that plays a major role in heart health and is also helpful in detoxifying many toxic chemicals and preventing asthma attacks. The author suggests supplementation with 1,000 milligrams a day for people with heart disease, asthma, or chemical sensitivity.

L-Glutamine

L-glutamine is the most common amino acid in the body. However, glutamine levels are often low during stress caused by illness, injury, or malnutrition. For elders with muscle wasting (sarcopenia), the author recommends taking 1,000 to 15,000 milligrams of glutamine daily in several doses throughout the day.

Several studies have reported that glutamine supplementation can increase the body's immunity to infection (Kim 2010). Several studies have reported that mixtures of the amino acids glutamine, arginine, and beta-hydroxy-beta-methylbutryrate (a leucine derivative) are useful in regaining muscle mass in patients who have lost much muscle mass due to malnutrition, cancer, or HIV infection (Clark 2000).

L-Arginine

L-arginine is another amino acid that plays a role in improving the body's immunity to infection and is helpful in building and

LUKE CURTIS, MD

maintaining muscle mass in elders (Kim 2010). For elders with muscle wasting (sarcopenia), the author recommends taking 1,000 to 15,000 milligrams of arginine daily in several doses throughout the day. High levels of arginine supplementation can lower blood pressure, which can be harmful to those who already have low blood pressure.

L-Leucine and Its Derivative Beta-Hydroxy-Beta-Methylbutyrate

Several studies have reported that beta-hydroxy-methylbutyrate (BHMB) helps to maintain muscle mass in elders and prevent muscle loss (sarcopenia) (Kim 2010).

SAMe or S-Adenosylmethionine

S-adenosylmethionine or SAMe is an amino acid derivative. Various studies have reported that supplementation with 100 milligrams of SAMe can be helpful in reducing depression and joint problems. SAMe is a fairly expensive supplement, so be sure to shop around for the best prices.

Omega-3 and Omega-6 Fatty Acids

Fats are comprised of long chains of carbon with hydrogen atoms attached and a carboxylic acid (COOH) group attached at the end. Carbon chains provide the backbone for fats and attached to each other by sharing electrons in a covalent bond. Some of the bonds between carbon chains of fat are single bonds, while some are double bonds. Fats in which all of the bonds are single are called saturated fats. Fats in which one of these carbon bonds is double are called monounsaturated fats, and fats in which more than the carbon bonds are double are called polyunsaturated fats. Fats in which the first double bond is present on the third carbon-carbon bond are called omega-3 fats. Fats in which the first double bond is present on the third carbon-carbon bond are called omega-6 fats. As noted in many chapters of this book, omega-3 fats have many health benefits and play many important roles in building and maintaining muscle and bone, fighting infection, heart disease, cancer, promoting good eye health, and reducing risk of depression and digestive problems.

Most double bonds of natural fats are arranged in an arrangement known as cis confirmation in which the chains point away from each other. However, treating unsaturated fats with heat and/or chemicals can produce a trans arrangement in which the double bonds form a U-shape with each other. Such trans fats are not found in large quantities in any unprocessed food. Trans fats are found in such foods as french fries, donuts, potato chips, and peanut butter and margarine prepared with hydrogenated vegetable oil. Consumption of trans fats have been linked to many health problems including higher rates of heart disease, hardening of the arteries, and acquiring Alzheimer's dementia (Kummerow 2009; Morris 2009). For more information about omega-3 and omega-6 fatty acids, please consult a biochemistry textbook or a Web site such as Wikipedia (Wikipedia 2010).

Omega-3 fat exists in several forms. Alpha-linolenic acid (ALA) has 18 carbon atoms and is found in many plant foods such as flax, soybean, canola, pumpkin, and walnut seeds and oils. Eicosapentaenoic acid (EPA) has 20 carbons, and docosahexaenoic acid (DHA) has 22 carbons. EPA and DHA are found in animal foods like fatty fish (salmon, mackerel, anchovies, sardines, and herring); fish oils; and grass-fed beef.

Research suggests that all three forms of omega-3 fats may be quite beneficial to health. The body is able to convert about 10% of the ALA to EPA, but only about 1% of the ALA to DHA (Brenna 2009). Therefore, folks obtaining their entire omega-3 fats from plant sources may be lacked in DHA. For best nutrition, it is good to consume omega-3 fats both in the ALA-rich plant form such from flax, soybean, canola, pumpkin, and walnut seeds/oils and in the DHA- and EPA-rich animal forms from fish, fish oils, or from grass-fed beef.

The following table lists omega-3 levels in common foods and oils. Please note that some common oils like corn, peanut, sunflower, and safflower oils have little or no omega-3 fatty acids. Table data from Whitney (2008), Dannenberger (2007), and Samman (2009).

Table: Omega-3 Content in Common Foods	
Food	Omega-3 Content in Grams
ANIMAL SOURCES	
Cod-liver oil, 1 tablespoon	3.0
Salmon oil, 1 tablespoon	2.8
Salmon, 3.5 ounces	1.4
Sardines, 3.5 ounces	1.2
Mackerel, Atlantic, 3.5 ounces	2.6
Herring, 3.5 ounces	1.8
Pollock, 3.5 ounces	0.5
Cod or haddock, 3.5 ounces	0.2
Feedlot beef, ground, 20% fat, 4 ounces	0.5
Grass-fed beef, ground, 20% fat, 4 ounces	1.3
Eggs, conventional, 1 large	0.1
Eggs, hens fed omega-3-enriched diets, 1 large	0.4
Butter, 1 tablespoon	0.4
PLANT SOURCES	
Flax seed oil, 1 tablespoon	8.5
Flax seeds, 1 ounce	5.6
Soybean oil, 1 tablespoon	1.0
Canola oil, 1 tablespoon	1.0
Pumpkin seeds, 1 ounce	2.4
Walnut oil, 1 tablespoon	1.6
Walnuts, 1 ounce	1.3
Corm oil, 1 tablespoon	0.0
Sunflower oil, 1 tablespoon	0.0
Safflower oil, 1 tablespoon	0.0
Peanut oil, 1 tablespoon	0.0

The author recommends that elders consume at least 4 grams of omega-3 fats daily. Most studies involving omega-3 fats and fatty acids involved consuming anywhere from 4 grams to 20 grams (about 1 to 4 teaspoons) of omega-3-rich fish, flax, or evening primrose oil. Many of the author's patients and friends consume only a 1 gram (1,000 milligram) capsule of fish oil daily, which is not enough for optimum health. As noted in chapter 17, cod liver or fish oil is generally much cheaper than the same oils in capsules. Try to see if you like the taste of various-flavored cod liver or fish oils on the market.

Omega-6 fats such as linoleic acid and arachidonic acid also play many important roles in human nutrition including formation of cell membranes, transport of fats, and providing energy (Whitney 2008). Corn, soy, safflower, sunflower, and walnut oils are particularly rich in omega-6 fats. However, most vegetable oils and the fat from meats and milk are rich in omega-6 acids, and anyone eating a diet with adequate fat is unlikely to be deficient in omega-6. Diets low in omega-3 fats but high in omega-3 fats have been associated with heart disease and other health problems (Whitney 2008).

Olive, peanut, and canola oils are rich in monounsaturated fats. Some studies have reported that diets high in monounsaturated fats such as the olive oil-rich Mediterranean Diet are associated with significantly lower rates of heart disease and stroke (Spence 2006).

VITAMINS. The following section will describe vitamins. Vitamins A, D, E, and K are fat soluble, while the B complex vitamins and vitamin C are water soluble.

Vitamin A

Vitamin A plays a key role in vision, immune system, reproduction, and child development and in building and maintaining tissue. Vitamin A is also an antioxidant that protects against oxidation damage to cells. Vitamin A comes in two forms, an animal form called retinol and a plant form called beta-carotene. Vitamin A is found in some animal sources like butter, cheese, milk, eggs, cod-liver oil, and fatty fish. Beta-carotene is found in many yellow and green vegetables such as carrots, pumpkins, sweet potatoes, broccoli, leaf lettuce, etc.

The US recommended daily allowance for vitamin A is 5,000 international units daily. The animal form or retinol is toxic in large doses. Consuming over 50,000 a day for years can cause side effects such as fatigue, appetite loss, nausea, dry skin, and brittle nails. Taking large amounts of vitamin A can also cause birth defects. It is probably best for pregnant women to consume no more than 10,000 international units per day of vitamin A. The plant or beta-carotene form of vitamin A is virtually nontoxic, although consuming over 100,000 international units daily of beta-carotene for long periods may cause the skin to turn orange (Murray 1996).

B VITAMINS

The following ten substances are part of the B vitamin family. All B vitamins are water soluble and play many important roles in many of the body's metabolic and energy-producing reactions. Many of these B vitamins are grouped together in "balanced" concentrations in vitamin supplements or B complex supplements.

Please note that brewer's yeast is an excellent source of most of the B vitamins, as well as protein and many minerals such as iron. However, allergies to brewer's yeast are fairly common. Brewer's yeast makes a wonderful nutritional supplement provided one is not allergic to the yeast. Special blends of brewer's yeast, which have a mild and pleasant flavor, are available in health food stores.

Thiamine (B$_1$)

Thiamine plays a key role in converting food into energy in the body and for mental functions. Thiamine is often extremely deficient in heavy alcohol drinkers and often causes severe mental problems in alcoholics. The richest sources of thiamine are food supplements, brewer's or baker's yeast, and wheat germ. Whole grains, peanuts, soybeans, sunflower seeds, and other nuts and beans are fair sources.

The recommended daily allowance for thiamine is 1.2 milligrams a day for men and 1.1 milligrams a day for women. The author recommends that 10 to 100 milligrams a day be consumed as supplements. High levels of thiamine (such as 8,000 milligrams a day) are virtually nontoxic. Alcoholics are often very deficient in thiamine and can experience severe neurological problems and even psychotic behavior as a result.

Riboflavin (B$_2$)

Riboflavin is another B vitamin critical for energy production, vision, production of blood, and health of mucous membranes such as the mouth and entire gastro-intestinal tract. The richest sources of riboflavin are supplements, brewer's and baker's yeast, and liver. Fair sources include many whole grains, nuts and seeds, and some vegetables such as mushrooms, kale, broccoli, and parsley.

The recommended daily allowance for riboflavin is 1.4 milligrams a day for men and 1.2 milligrams a day for women. The author recommends that at least 10 milligrams a day of riboflavin be consumed as supplements (Murray 1996). Large amounts of riboflavin are virtually nontoxic.

LUKE CURTIS, MD

Niacin (B$_3$)

Niacin is a vitamin essential for energy production, regulation of blood sugar and cholesterol, and in antioxidation and detoxification reactions. The richest sources of niacin include brewer's and baker's yeast, whole wheat and whole rice, liver, and sunflower and sesame seeds. In the late nineteenth and early twentieth century, a number of people in the United States lived mainly on corn, a grain low in niacin. They developed a niacin-deficiency disease called pellagra, which involves diarrhea, dementia, and dermatitis (irritated skin).

The recommended daily allowance of niacin is 15 milligrams a day for adults. The author recommends elders consume at least 50 milligrams a day of niacin. Much larger amounts (100 to 10,000 milligrams daily) are often given in patients trying to lower the levels of LDL ("bad") cholesterol and triglycerides in the blood (please see chapter 8 for more about the LDL cholesterol-lowering properties of niacin). High levels of niacin can cause unpleasant skin flushing in some people. Persons prescribed niacin for lowering LDL cholesterol should start at a low dose of 100 milligrams a day and gradually build up the dose to 1,000 milligrams a day or higher as needed to control LDL cholesterol. Very high levels of niacin (over 1,000 milligrams a day) can also impair the body's blood sugar regulation mechanism, so diabetics should probably not consume more than 100 or 200 milligrams a day of niacin (Murray 1996).

Pyridoxine (B$_6$)

Pyridoxine is important for many functions including the synthesis of blood and other proteins; maintaining the heart, blood vessels, and immune system; and manufacturing hormones and chemical transmitters for the nervous system. Supplementation with pyridoxine has been helpful for preventing or controlling a wide range of health problems including autism, asthma, heart disease, depression, diabetes, premenstrual syndrome, carpal tunnel syndrome, and low levels of red blood cells (anemia). Good sources of pyridoxine include supplements, brewer's and baker's yeast, whole grains, soybeans, walnuts, beans and lentils, bananas, and green vegetables like broccoli and spinach.

The recommended daily allowance for pyridoxine for adults over age 70 years is 1.7 milligrams a day for men and 1.5 milligrams a day for women. The author recommends that all elders consume a supplement containing at least 10 milligrams of pyridoxine daily. Doses of 50 to 100 milligrams a day are often prescribed for many health conditions such as anemia and are considered quite safe. Consuming very high levels of pyridoxine (over 2,000 milligrams a day) for several months have been associated with nerve problems such as tingling sensation in the feet and loss of muscle coordination (Murray 1996).

Cobalmin (B$_{12}$)

Cobalmin or vitamin B$_{12}$ is involved in manufacturing red blood cells and in maintaining structures of the nervous system. The richest sources of vitamin B$_{12}$ are supplements, liver, kidneys, clams, oysters, fish, eggs, and dairy products. Cobalmin is found in significant quantities only in animal foods, so that strict vegetarians (vegans) need to take a supplement of vitamin B$_{12}$. Sometimes cobalmin is given to patients by injection, but that is not absolutely necessary.

The US recommended daily allowance for cobalmin is 2.4 micrograms per day. About 40% of all elders are deficient in vitamin B$_{12}$ (Lindenbaum 1994). Absorption of vitamin B$_{12}$ in the intestines often becomes less efficient with age. Deficiencies of B$_{12}$ can cause low red blood cell counts (anemia) and many neurological problems. Cobalmin has little toxicity, with quantities of up to 2,000 micrograms (2 milligrams) a day being taken for years without ill effects (Murray 1996). The author recommends that all seniors take supplements containing at least 50 micrograms per day of cobalmin (vitamin B_{12}).

Folate

Folate (also known as folic acid) has many vital functions in the body including the synthesis of all new cells including red blood cells, developing and maintaining a healthy nervous system, and promoting heart and bone health. The richest sources of folate are brewer's yeast, wheat germ, beans, and green vegetables such as spinach, asparagus, and broccoli. Various studies have reported that folate supplementation can reduce risk of hardening of the arteries (atherosclerosis), bone loss (osteoporosis), and depression. Supplementation of 1,000 micrograms of folate daily to pregnant women is also associated with significantly lower rates of neural tube defects (such as spina bifida) in newborn children (Murray 1996). To prevent neural tube defects, all sexually active women of reproductive age should take at least 1,000 micrograms of folate daily.

The recommended daily allowance of folate is 400 micrograms daily. Folate is a safe supplement, although some studies have reported higher rates of nausea and flatulence when consuming 10,000 or more micrograms per day (Murray 1996). The author recommends that elders take at least 400 micrograms a day of supplemental folate daily.

Biotin

Biotin is a B vitamin that functions in the manufacture and metabolism of fats and amino acids. The best diet sources of biotin are brewer's yeast, cheese, liver, and soybeans. Raw egg whites contain avidin, a protein that prevents biotin absorption. Eggs should always be consumed cooked and never raw.

Bacteria in the intestines can also manufacture biotin. Biotin supplementation can be useful for diabetics, those with dandruff, and those with skin and nail problems (Murray 1996). The recommended daily allowance of biotin is 30 micrograms daily for adults over age 70. The author recommends that seniors take a supplement containing at least 300 micrograms a day of biotin. Doses of 3,000 micrograms a day for many years have been administered with no apparent ill health effects (Murray 1996).

Pantothenic Acid

Pantothenic acid, or vitamin B_5, is involved in the manufactured of coenzyme A and acyl-carrier protein, which are involved in energy production and the manufacture of red blood cells and hormones. Pantothenic acid is found in brewer's yeast, liver, peanuts, mushrooms, and many other whole foods. The recommended daily allowance of patothenic acid is 5 milligrams a day. The author recommends that elders consume 50 milligrams a day of pantothenic acid. No adverse health effects of taking pantothenic acid have been reported (Murray 1996).

Choline

Choline is an "unofficial" member of the B vitamins. Choline is essential for manufacturing neurotransmitter chemicals and the main components of our cell membranes such as phosphatidylcholine (lecithin). Choline is found in large quantities in liver and other meats, in eggs, and in peanuts and peanut butter. Some research suggests that supplementation with phosphatidylcholine can be helpful for liver disorders, bipolar depression, and Alzheimer's disease (Murray 1996). The recommended daily allowance for choline in adults over 70 years is 550 milligrams for men and 425 milligrams for women. Choline doses of up to 10,000 milligrams daily are believed to be safe.

LUKE CURTIS, MD

Inositol

Inositol is another "unofficial" B vitamin that plays a role in building cell membranes. Inositol is found in many plant foods such as citrus fruits, whole grains, nuts, seeds, and legumes (beans). Inositol may play a vital role in helping to prevent cancer, diabetes, depression, and heart attacks.

Vitamin C Ascorbate

Vitamin C is a water-soluble vitamin and a strong antioxidant. Vitamin C plays an important role in supporting immunity from infection and in building and maintaining body tissue. Vitamin C also plays a vital role in preventing heart disease and cancer and can reduce the severity of asthma and the common cold (Murray 1996).

Vitamin C is found in many fruits and vegetables including citrus fruits (oranges, grapefruit, lemons, and limes); melons; kiwi; tomatoes; potatoes; peppers; broccoli; cabbage; and parsley. Vitamin C is a rather fragile vitamin. Cooking fruits and vegetables or storing cut fruits and vegetables in the air for several days can significantly reduce vitamin C levels (Murray 1996). For maximum levels of vitamin C, be sure to eat fruits and vegetables within a couple of hours of cutting them open.

During the fifteenth through eighteenth centuries, many thousands of sailors on long voyages became very sick and died of a vitamin C deficiency diet called scurvy. The lack of fresh fruits and vegetables on long ship journeys caused scurvy. From 1753 to 1771, British naval surgeon James Lind and British naval captain James Cook discovered that citrus fruits like oranges, grapefruit, lemons, and limes could completely prevent scurvy (All Experts 2010). British sailors were then frequently called "limeys" since they always carried citrus fruit on long voyages to prevent scurvy. This discovery saved the lives of many thousands of sailors and sea travelers. The author's great-grandfather talked about taking along oranges on their four-week voyage from Hamburg to New York when immigrating to the United States in 1853.

The recommended daily allowance of vitamin C for adults over 70 years is 90 milligrams for men and 75 milligrams for women. Most studies have suggested that 500 to 2,000 milligrams a day is a good supplemental dose of vitamin C (Murray 1996). The cost of vitamin C varies greatly, so be sure to shop around for best prices.

Vitamin C is almost nontoxic in patients with normal kidney function. Doses up to 20 grams a day have virtually no adverse health effects (Murray 1996). However, large quantities of vitamin C can cause diarrhea (Natural Cures 2010).

Dialysis patients are often very low in vitamin C since they can lose several hundred milligrams of vitamin C in each dialysis session (Handelman 2007). However, excessive vitamin C can cause toxic buildup of oxalate in bloodstream and kidneys (Handelman 2007). Intake of up to 500 mg a day of vitamin C by dialysis patients is believed to be safe (Keven 2003). A recent study of hemodialysis patients reported that consumption of 200 milligrams of supplemental vitamin C daily was associated with preventing vitamin C deficiency in nearly all dialysis patients without producing a toxic buildup of vitamin C or oxalate (Fehrman-Ekholm 2008). For more information about supplements for kidney failure patients, please see chapter 14 on kidney failure.

Vitamin D

Vitamin D is another fat-soluble vitamin that plays a key role in bone growth and maintenance, immunity against infection, and protection against cancer, heart disease, and autoimmune diseases like type 1 diabetes. Vitamin D is found in only a few foods such as fatty fish and fish oils, eggs, and fortified milk.

LUKE CURTIS, MD

Milk is fortified with about 400 international units of vitamin D per quart, while cod-liver oil contains about 1,300 international units of vitamin D per tablespoon, and fatty fish like salmon, herring, mackerel, or sardines contain about 300 international units of D per 4-ounce serving (Stechschulte 2009). Vitamin D can also be made from cholesterol in body if the skin is exposed to sunlight.

Vitamin D deficiency is very common. In recent years, use of sunscreen to reduce skin cancer risk has also increased risk of vitamin D deficiency (Stechshulte 2009). Vitamin D deficiency is more common in older persons, dark-skinned people, and people who live far from the equator as compared to younger persons, light-skinned people, or people who live near the equator. Vitamin D deficiency is very common in elders. One huge study of 3,170 US adults over age 60 years reported that vitamin D deficiency was found in 76% of whites, 96% of blacks, and 92% of Mexican Americans! (Ginde 2009).

The US recommended daily allowance for vitamin D is only 400 international units per day. Many researchers suggest that this limit should be raised to at least 800 international units daily (Stechschulte 2009). The author urges that all seniors who do not get heavy sun exposure to consume 800 to 2,000 international units of vitamin D daily in foods such as vitamin D fortified milk, cod-liver oil, and vitamin D supplements. A review of twenty studies reported that high dose vitamin D supplements (700 international units a day or more) reduced bone breaks in elderly by 23%, but lower dose vitamin D (400 international units a day) did not reduce rates of bone fractures in elders (Bischoff 2009).

Vitamin D supplements are quite safe in reasonable doses. Numerous studies have given patients 5,000 to 18,000 international units of vitamin D daily for years with no reported health problems or changes in calcium metabolism (Hathcock 2007). Vitamin D can be toxic if taken in huge quantities. Some studies have reported that supplemental levels of 100,000 or more international units a day for periods of months to years can interfere with calcium metabolism (Hathcock 2007).

Vitamin E

Vitamin E is vitamin with many antioxidation properties that protect cells from damage from oxidation. Vitamin E is essential for wound healing, maintaining immunity, fighting infection, reproduction, heart health, fighting cancer, preventing autoimmune diseases like lupus, and many other functions. The best sources of vitamin E are polyunsaturated vegetable oils, nuts, seeds like sunflower and pumpkin seeds, and whole grains (especially wheat germ). Numerous studies show that higher consumption of vitamin E (in food or supplements) is associated with significantly lower rates of heart disease (Murray 1996).

Vitamin E is available in several chemical forms including d-alpha-tocopherol, d-alpha-tocopherol avetate, d-alpha-tocopherol succinate, d-beta-tocopherol, d-gamma-tocopherol, and d-alpha-tcoctrienol. The best supplement forms contain a mixture of these forms of vitamin E. Synthetic vitamin E usually contains only d-alpha-tocopherol, which is not as potent as the mixed tocopherols (Murray1996).

The recommended daily allowance for vitamin E is 30 international units daily. Consuming a lot of oil and other fats increases the body's need for vitamin E. Vitamin E appears to be a safe vitamin, with intakes up to 3,200 international units daily for years having no obvious reported side effects (Murray 1996). On the other hand, one study that analyzed death rates in a number of studies reported that high consumption of vitamin E supplements may be harmful. As compared to persons who took no supplements, death rates were slightly lower among patients who took 30 to 150 international units per day and were slightly higher in those who took 400 of more international units of vitamin E daily (Miller 2005). The author would recommend that most

LUKE CURTIS, MD

adults consume 100 to 200 international units of vitamin E daily, until further research determines the best dose to take.

Vitamin K

Vitamin K is a fat-soluble vitamin. Vitamin K is found in many green vegetables such as leaf lettuce, parsley, broccoli, cabbage, and green tea. Vitamin K is also produced by intestinal bacteria. Vitamin K is necessary for the blood clotting and for proper bone formation.

Vitamin K deficiency is rare in folks eating green vegetables. Few adverse side effects have been reported by getting large amounts of vitamin K in food and supplements. However, eating large amounts of green vegetables can reduce the effect of certain blood-thinning drugs like coumaden. Patients on blood-thinning drugs like coumaden should eat consistent amounts of green vegetables every day so their dosages of blood thinner can be adjusted accordingly. If patients on blood-thinning drugs abruptly eat large amounts of green vegetables, they may get too much vitamin K, which can promote too much blood clotting (i.e., make the blood too "thick"). If patients on blood thinning abruptly stop eating green vegetables for several days, they may get too little vitamin K, which can make it too hard for the blood to clot (i.e., make the blood too "thin").

Coenzyme Q_{10}

Coenzyme Q_{10} is also known as ubiquinone and is essential for energy-producing reactions in the mitochondria of the cells. The mitochondria are organelles in the cells that are responsible for most of the body's energy-producing reactions. Small amounts of coenzyme Q_{10} are present in most whole foods. While some coenzyme Q_{10} can be produced in the body, many people are deficient of coenzyme Q_{10} and must take more of it in the diet. Various studies have reported that supplementation with coenzyme Q_{10} is useful for people with chronic fatigue, heart attacks, heart failure, diabetes, and kidney failure (Murray 1996).

Many elders are prescribed statin drugs (Lipitor, Zocor) to lower LDL cholesterol levels. While these statin drugs are very effective at lowering LDL cholesterol, they possess some bad side effects including muscle weakness and pain and significantly lower coenzyme Q_{10} levels. Supplementation with 100 milligrams daily of coenzyme Q_{10} or more is highly recommended to all patients taking statin drugs. One New York study reported that 100 milligrams of supplemental coenzyme Q_{10} daily significantly reduced muscle pain and weakness in eighteen patients with statin related muscle problems (Caso 2007).

Coenzyme Q_{10} is a very safe supplement, with doses of 300 to 1,000 milligrams being consumed daily with no know adverse health effects of interactions with other drugs. The author recommends that all heart patients, chronic fatigue patients, and patients taking LDL cholesterol-lowering statin drugs consume 100 milligrams or more of coenzyme Q_{10} daily. Prices of coenzyme Q_{10} vary widely, so be sure to shop around for the best price.

Glucosamine and Chondroitin Sulfate

Glucosamine sulfate and chondroitin sulfate compounds are found in healthy joint tissue and often become depleted in osteoarthritis patients. Glucosamine and chrondroitin can be manufactured by humans from other dietary components, but research has indicated that older people manufacture significantly less of these compounds than younger people. Various studies have reported that daily supplementation with 1,500 milligrams or more of glucosamine and 800 milligrams or more of chondroitin sulfate can significantly reduce joint pain, stiffness, and joint narrowing in patients with osteoarthritis (Richy 2003).

It takes several months for the maximum benefits of glucosamine and chondroitin sulfate, so do not be discouraged if you do see results in the first few weeks. Be sure to shop around for the best prices of glucosamine and chondroitin sulfate.

MINERALS

Calcium

Calcium is very common mineral that comprises about 2% of our bodies. Calcium is involved with bone growth and many other reactions including controlling heartbeat. Sufficient vitamin D is required for proper metabolism of calcium. Calcium and vitamin D supplementation has been associated with greater bone mass and fewer bone fractures in osteoporosis patients. A meta-analysis of twenty-nine studies of 63,897 adults older than 50 years reported that consumption of 800 to 1,500 milligrams of calcium and 400 to 800 international units of vitamin D was associated with an overall statistically significant 12% reduction in osteoporosis fractures (Tang 2007).

Calcium is found in milk, yogurt, cheese, dark green vegetables like broccoli, mustard, greens, and parsley and in fish eaten with bones such as canned salmon and sardines.

Calcium is also found in a number of supplements such as calcium citrate, calcium carbonate, and calcium joined (chelated) with protein. Calcium is absorbed in the intestines most efficiently in calcium citrate or chelated forms as compared to the calcium carbonate form (Murray 1996). Avoid calcium supplements containing dolomite or bone meal since they sometimes can be contaminated with toxic lead (Murray 1996).

The recommended daily allowance for calcium is 1,200 milligrams a day for adults over aged 70 years (Whitney 2008). The average US adult over age 60 years consumes only about 60% of this minimum daily requirement (Park 2008). The author recommends that elders consume at least 500 milligrams of calcium daily and at least 1,000 milligrams daily if they do not consume dairy products.

Magnesium

Magnesium is another common mineral involved in over 500 chemical reactions. Magnesium is found in a number of foods such as soybeans, other legumes, seeds, nuts, and leafy green vegetables. Organically grown foods tend to be higher in magnesium than foods grown with chemical fertilizers (Murray 1996). Many studies have shown that magnesium supplementation can be useful for many conditions including heart disease, high blood pressure, headaches, asthma, and chronic fatigue/fibromyalgia (Murray 1996).

The recommended daily allowance for magnesium is 420 milligrams a day for men and 320 milligrams a day for women. Average magnesium consumption among women over 65 years is only 68% of the USRDA (Rude 2009). The author recommends that all elders take at least 400 milligrams of supplemental magnesium daily. High consumption of magnesium (over 2,000 milligrams a day) can cause diarrhea.

Phosphorus

Phosphorus is involved with bone growth and many of the body's energy-producing reactions. Phosphorus is found in many foods such as milk, meat, fish, and whole grains.

The US recommended daily allowance for phosphorus is 700 milligrams per day. Deficiencies of phosphorus are rare in those who eat a well-balanced diet. Huge amounts of supplemental phosphorus can reduce calcium absorption (Whitney 2008).

Potassium

Potassium is another common mineral in the body that plays vital role in controlling fluid balance in the body, maintaining nerve impulses and plays a role in enzyme reactions.

Potassium is found in many foods such as fruits, vegetables and dairy products. Citrus fruits, squash, artichoke, tomatoes, soybeans and other beans, bananas, and potatoes are especially rich in potassium (Whitney 2008). Many studies have reported that consumption of potassium-rich fruits and vegetables are effective at controlling high blood pressure (Alonso 2004). For a fuller discussion of the blood pressure-lowering effects of consuming fruits, vegetables, and potassium, please see the section on high blood pressure in chapter 8.

The recommended daily allowance (RDA) for potassium is 4,700 milligrams a day for adults. Studies involving elderly adults have reported that average intake of potassium is only about 50% of USRDA (Gorelik 2003). The author recommends that all seniors consume at least five servings (one-half cup) of a wide range of fruits and vegetables daily plus at least three servings of dairy products in order to get sufficient intake of potassium. Potassium supplements may be useful for people who cannot eat sufficient fruits and vegetables.

High potassium intakes can be harmful for those with kidney failure. The author urges all kidney patients to consult a nutritionist or nutrition-minded physician or nurse for advice on potassium consumption.

Sodium

Sodium is found in common table salt. Sodium plays an important role in maintaining water balance and blood pressure. Sodium is added to many prepared foods such as meats, soups, tomato juice, TV dinners, breads, and snack foods. Salt is also often added to food like meat and vegetables at the table.

The recommended level of sodium consumption for adults over age 70 is between 1,200 and 2,300 milligrams a day (Whitney 2008). Many adults consume over 5,000 milligrams of sodium daily (Karppanen 2006) Limiting sodium intake can be helpful for those with high blood pressure (Karppanen 2006). For a fuller description of the effects of lowering sodium on blood pressure, please see chapter 8.

Deficiencies in sodium and chloride are rare in persons taking adequate salt in diet. Sodium sometimes is low in people who experience heavy sweating, vomiting, or diarrhea, and people with these conditions need to consume water and sodium to make up for these losses (Whitney 2008).

People who deliberately limit their sodium intake may also be low in sodium. Please see chapter 15 for discussion of low sodium and low blood pressure on chronic fatigue.

Chloride

Chloride is found in common table salt or sodium chloride. Chloride plays an important role in maintaining water balance in the body. Chloride also helps form hydrochloride acid in the stomach that is required to digest food.

Chloride deficiencies are rare among people getting sufficient salt in the diet. Chloride may become deficient in people who experience vomiting, diarrhea, and heavy sweating (Whitney 2008).

Iron

Iron is an important component of hemoglobin in the red blood cells. Hemoglobin transports oxygen and carbon dioxide in the blood and gives blood its red color.

Iron also plays a role in many important enzymatic reactions. The richest food sources of iron are kelp and other sea vegetables, brewer's yeast, pumpkin and sunflower seeds, whole grains, nuts, meat, eggs, dried fruit like prunes, and dark green vegetables like parsley and broccoli. The iron in animal sources like meat and eggs is generally better absorbed than the iron in plant sources (Whitney 2008).

The recommended daily allowance of iron is 8 milligrams a day for adults over age 70 years. About 10% of the US population over 65 years suffers from iron deficiency anemia (Guralnik 2005). Elders should have their blood tested at least every two or three years for hemoglobin and iron levels. If their blood levels of iron and hemoglobin are normal, they probably will not need an iron supplement. If elders are low in hemoglobin and/iron stores, the author recommends that they consume 15 to 45 milligrams of supplemental iron daily. Remember that many other nutrients are needed to build up red blood cells including protein and B complex vitamins like folate and vitamin B_{12}.

High consumption of iron for long periods may cause iron overload in the blood and increase risk of heart and liver problems (Whitney 2008).

For a discussion on treatment of anemia in kidney failure patients, please see diet and supplements section in chapter 14.

Zinc

Zinc is a mineral required for the function of over two hundred enzymes in the body and plays a role with many hormones including insulin, thyroid hormone, and growth hormone. Zinc is required for proper function of the eyes, growth, sleep, immune function, sexual function, wound healing, and prevention of depression and dementia (Murray 2006). Many chapters of this book discuss the benefits of zinc in more detail. The best food source of zinc by far is oysters. Other good sources of zinc are other shellfish like shrimp, fish, red meats, and whole grains, nuts, and legumes grown on soil with sufficient zinc.

The recommended daily allowance (RDA) of zinc is 15 milligrams per day. Studies involving elderly adults have reported that average intake of zinc is only about 60% of USRDA (Prasad 1993). The author recommends that all elders obtain at least 15 to 30 milligrams of zinc in supplements daily. Some authorities recommend as much as 80 milligrams of supplemental zinc daily to prevent macular degeneration (Raniga 2009).

Prolonged intakes of zinc (more than 250 milligrams a day) can cause toxic effects such as anemia (low concentration of red blood cells), lowered levels of HDL ("good") cholesterol, and depressed immune function. Too much zinc in the diet can reduce the intestinal absorption of copper (Murray 1996).

Copper

Copper is important for many energy-producing reactions, for making red blood cells and many proteins such as collagen and for eye health. Copper is found in a number of foods such as oysters, shellfish, sea vegetables, fish, legumes, and chocolate.

The recommended daily allowance of copper is 0.9 milligrams a day for adults. Copper deficiency is fairly common in elders, especially those who are malnourished or tube fed (Curtis 2008). The author recommends that elders consume 1 to 2 milligrams of copper daily. Too much copper in the diet can reduce the intestinal absorption of zinc. Copper supplementation of over 100 milligrams per day can cause nausea and vomiting. Liver damage is also possible for those consuming over 100 milligrams a day of copper for long periods. A few genetic disorders like Wilson's disease can cause toxic accumulation of copper in the body (Whitney 2008; Murray 1996).

LUKE CURTIS, MD

Chromium

Chromium is essential for a molecule called glucose tolerance factor that the body uses to help control blood sugar. Glucose tolerance factor is especially useful for controlling blood sugar in diabetics. A number of studies have reported that taking 200 to 100 micrograms daily of supplemental chromium (in the chromium picolinate form) is useful for controlling blood sugar in diabetics (Nahas 2009). The best diet sources of chromium are brewer's yeast, meats, and whole grains.

The recommended daily allowance for chromium is only 30 micrograms daily for men and 20 micrograms daily for women over 70 years (Whitney 2008). Many experts feel these chromium intake levels are far too low and should be raised to at least 200 micrograms a day of chromium (Murray,1996). The majority of elders consume less than 50 micrograms of chromium daily (Vaquero 2002). The author recommends that all elders take a chromium supplement of at least 200 micrograms daily and all diabetics take at least 400 micrograms of supplemental chromium daily.

Note: All supplements provide chromium its trivalent chemical form such as chromium picolinate. The hexavalent chemical form is used by industry and is a proven cancer-causing chemical (carcinogen) (Murray 1996).

Selenium

Selenium is an antioxidant element that protects cells from oxidative damage and plays a role in several enzyme reactions. Many studies have linked higher levels of selenium consumption with lower levels of heart disease and cancer and increased immunity to infection (Flores-Mateo 2006; Jacobs 2004; Etminan 2005; Wintergerest 2007). Good food sources of selenium include whole grains, Brazil nuts, and vegetables grown in soil with sufficient selenium.

The recommended daily allowance for selenium is 55 micrograms a day. Most adults over age 65 years consume less than 55 micrograms of selenium a day (Vaquero 2002). The author suggests that 75 to 100 micrograms is a good supplementation levels for elders. Levels of selenium above 1,000 micrograms day for prolonged periods can produce toxic effects like fatigue, brittle hair and nails, and garlic breath odor (Whitney 2008).

Manganese

Manganese is a trace metal needed for growth and repair of muscle and bone and for control of carbohydrate and fat metabolism. Good sources of manganese are nuts, whole grains, and leafy vegetables grown on soil with adequate manganese. The official daily requirement for manganese is 2.3 milligrams per day for men and 1.8 milligrams per day for women. Supplements of 5 to 15 milligrams per day are sometimes taken in diabetic patients and patients with sprain injuries. High levels of manganese (more than 100 milligrams per day) can cause nervous system disorders (Whitney 2008).

Boron

Boron is a trace element that may be helpful in building and maintaining bone, cartilage, and joints. The many dietary sources of boron are fruits and vegetables grown on boron-rich soil. There is no recommended daily level of boron in the diet. Patients with bone loss and joint problems often take 3 to 9 milligrams of boron per day. Supplementation of boron at levels exceeding 500 milligrams per day can cause nausea, diarrhea, and vomiting (Murray 1996).

LUKE CURTIS, MD

Iodine

Iodine is essential for thyroid hormone function. Iodine is found in ocean fish, seaweeds such as kelp, and supplements. The recommended daily allowance of iodine is 150 micrograms per day. The author recommends that all elders either consume sea vegetables and fish regularly and/or get an iodine supplement containing 150 to 500 micrograms per day. Some studies have been reported that high levels of iodine supplementation (750 to 250,000 micrograms per day) can reduce thyroid hormone secretion and cause acnelike symptoms (Murray 1996).

Strontium

Strontium is found in small quantities in many foods like milk and vegetables. There is no recommended daily allowance for strontium. As noted in chapter 5, daily supplements of 2,000 milligrams of strontium daily can significantly improve bone mass and reduce risk of bone breaks in elders with osteoporosis (Meunier 2004).

Silicon

Silicon is a very common mineral with about 25% of the earth's crust consisting of silicon. In the body, it is present in small amounts. Whole grains and root vegetables like beets, carrots, and potatoes are rich sources of silicon. The exact function of silicon in the body is not well known. Many researchers feel that silicon may play a role in bone, tooth, nail, and cartilage formation (Murray 1996).

Fluoride

Fluoride is needed in small amounts for healthy teeth and bones. The main sources of fluoride are fish, tea, fluoridated water, and toothpaste with fluoride. Too much fluoride can damage teeth. Many water supplies have about 0.5 to 1.0 milligram of fluoride added per liter (1.1 quarts). The recommended daily allowance for fluoride is 3.1 milligrams per day for men and 3.1 milligrams a day for women. The suggested upper limit for fluoride consumption is 10 milligrams a day. People drinking fluoridated water are unlikely to be deficient in fluoride (Whitney 2008).

Vanadium

Vanadium is a metal that participates in enzymes involved with control of hormones, cholesterol, and blood sugar. The best food sources of vanadium are buckwheat, soy, oats, dill, black pepper, parsley, and shellfish like shrimp and lobster. Diabetics and bodybuilders occasionally take vanadium as a supplement. Supplement levels of 10 to 100 micrograms a day appear to be safe. Cramping and diarrhea has been reported in humans who take 22 to 100 micrograms per day (Murray 1996).

Molybdenum

Molybdenum is a metal involved in several enzyme reactions. Molybdenum is found in legumes, nuts, whole grains, milk, and leafy green vegetables. The minimum daily requirement is 50 micrograms per day. Molybdenum deficiency is rare in those getting a well-balanced diet (Whitney 2008).

Probiotic Bacteria and Yeasts

Probiotics include "friendly" bacteria like *Lactobacillus* and *Bifidobacterium* and "friendly" yeasts like *Saccharomyces*. As noted in chapter 7 on hospital nutrition and chapter 14 on digestive disorders, the use of oral probiotics organisms can reduce risk of infections in the digestive and genital tracts and can reduce symptoms of irritable bowel disease. Probiotics also produce important nutrients like vitamin K and some B vitamins in the gut (Murray 1996).

At present, it is not certain which types of probiotics bacteria and yeast are most effective. Common probiotic bacteria including many species of *Lactobacillus* including *acidophilus*, *bulgaricus casei*, *fermentum*, *plantarum*, and *brevis*, several strains of *Bifidobacterium*, and *Streptococcus thermophilus*. The common probiotic yeast is *Saccharomyces boulardii*. Probiotics are believed to be safe in persons with normal immune systems, although *Saccharomyces* has occasionally caused bad infections in those with compromised immune systems such as HIV/AIDS patients (Enache-Angouvant 2005). Much more research on probiotic bacteria and yeasts is needed to determine which strains or probiotic bacteria and yeasts have optimum disease fighting and health promoting properties.

The richest source of probiotic bacteria and yeasts are available in capsule form in the health food or drug store. Such probiotics have to be kept in the refrigerator until used. Plan on taking enough probiotic capsules to get 1 to 10 billion live (viable) bacteria or yeasts per day. Mixtures of several types of probiotic bacteria may be more effective than just one type. Probiotics are also often given to tube-fed patients to prevent infections from *Clostridium difficile* and other severe intestinal infections (DeLegge 2008). Most yogurts also contain live (viable) bacteria, but total counts vary considerably from several million to several billion viable bacteria per cup of yogurt (Baroja 2007).

Some carbohydrates like lactose (from milk) and inulin (from Jerusalem artichokes) stimulate growth of helpful bacteria like *Lactobacillus* and *Bifidobacterium*. Such carbohydrates are called "prebiotics" and are being increasingly consumed by health conscious people. On the other hand, diets high in refined sugars can stimulate overgrowth of yeasts in the intestine.

Probiotics and prebiotics can improve the bacteria in the intestines. Many studies have reported that supplementing adults over age 65 years with probiotic bacteria like *Lactobacillus* or *Bifidobacterium* (with or without prebiotics like inulin) results in significantly higher intestinal levels of good bacteria like *Lactobacillus* and *Bifidobacterium* and significantly lower levels of harmful organisms like *Candida* (a yeast) (Tiihonen 2009).

Probiotics are especially recommended for elders who have undergone numerous courses of antibiotics. Oral antibiotics kill off good bacteria and encourage growth of harmful bacteria like *Closteridium difficile* and harmful yeasts like *Candida*. Use of probiotic helpful bacteria like *Lactobacillus* and *Bifidobacterium* can help restore the intestines to good health (Tiihonen 2009).

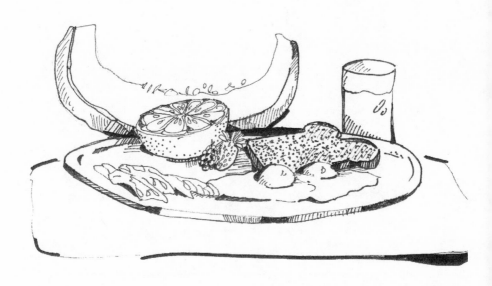

CHAPTER 19

MENU SUGGESTIONS FOR ELDERS

The following list gives some ideas for healthy menus for elders. These diets may have to be altered somewhat if the senior has food allergies or religious proscriptions against certain foods. Calorie levels may also have to altered to maintain a healthy weight. For adequate supply of water, elders should drink at least 6 eight ounce glasses of water, milk, juice, coffee, tea etc during the day. More fluids may be needed in hot weather or if the senior sweats profusely.

Breakfast Ideas

Breakfast should always include a good source of complete protein such as meat, fish, egg, cheese or milk. Breakfast is also a good time to get one to three servings of fruits and vegetables and a serving of milk or cheese.

- Omelets and other Egg Dishes—one or two eggs provide an inexpensive source of protein and many other nutrients. Other nutritious items can be easily added to omelets such as milk, cheese, yogurt, meat, kelp and many vegetables such as onions, peppers, broccoli, parsley, tomatoes, carrots etc.

- Meat or Fish—Many kinds of meat and fish are suitable for breakfast. If you like bacon, Canadian bacon contains less fat than the standard bacon strips. Turkey sausage contains less fat than standard sausage. High protein soy based breakfast "sausage" and "links" are available.

- Cereals. Should always be whole grain. May be eaten either hot or cold. Hot cereals such as oatmeal are often considerably cheaper than prepared cereals like shredded wheat. Prepared cold cereals are generally fairly expensive in supermarkets, however coupons and/or sales can often reduce cost of cold cereals.

  Nuts, seeds, and many kinds of fresh fruit and berries can be added to fresh fruit to add both flavor and nutrition. Adding soy grits (also known as textured vegetable protein) can boost protein since soy grits are 50% high quality protein.

  Avoid donuts, sweet rolls and other pastries. Most of them are loaded with sugar and many of them are loaded with unhealthful trans fats.

- Bread or Toast. If eaten should be whole grain. For spreads butter or peanut butter as preferable to trans-fat containing margarines.

- Fresh Fruits—Fresh fruit is preferable to fruit juice since whole fruits contain fiber and many phytochemicals lacking in fruit juice. Oranges, grapefruits, bananas, grapes, blueberries, blackberries, raspberries, strawberries, serviceberries, pineapple, cantaloupe, honeydew and watermelon are all excellent fresh fruits for breakfast.

LUKE CURTIS, MD

- Beverages. For drinks, milk, yogurt, coffee, tea, tomato juice or V-8, fruit juice are good choices.

- Breakfast is also a good time to take supplements such as pills, tablets and fish/ cod liver oil.

Lunch Ideas

- Lunch is a good time for soup. Soups can be prepared with a white range of nutritious ingredients including meat, fish, beans, lentils, whole grains and a wide range of vegetables such as potatoes, carrots, parsley, peas, leeks, cabbage and onions. To save time, large amounts of soup can be prepared and portions can be frozen and reheated for later use.

- Both lunch and dinner are good times for salads. Prepare salads with a wide range of vegetables and fruits. *Use your imagination when preparing salads!* Lettuce, parsley, dandelion greens, sprouts (alfalfa, onion, radish, broccoli), onions, tomatoes, broccoli, bok choi, cucumbers and fruits are great in salads. For omega 3 fats, eat salads with small amounts of dressing prepared with flax, soybean, walnut or canola oils.

- Cooked Vegetables—Vegetables may be easily cooked in a pot with a metal steamer.

- Meat or Fish. Try to eat at least a 3 ounce serving of meat or fish at both the midday and evening meals. For omega 3 fats and iodine, try to eat fish at least 2 times a week. Many supermarkets often prepared meats and fish which are easy to heat and serve. Meat patties made from beef, chicken, turkey or salmon are also very easy to heat and serve.

- Whole grain breads.

- Desserts—Fresh fruits, nuts, seeds, sugar free ice cream or cakes and pies prepared with sugar substitutes like Stevia.

- Water, milk, yogurt, vegetable juice, coffee, tea. Avoid sweetened colas and alcohol.

Supper Ideas

- Soup—Please see lunch section above.
- Salad—Please see salad section above.
- Meat or fish. Please see section above.
- Whole grain breads

- Cooked vegetables—Such as corn, broccoli, mustard greens, spinach, green beans, brussels sprouts. To fight cancer. try to eat cruciferous vegetables like broccoli, cauliflower, brussels sprouts, cabbage, bok choi or radish at least 3 times weekly.

  Avoid fried vegetables like french fries and onion rings which contain unhealthful trans fats.

- Sweet Potatoes and White Potatoes. Can be fixed in a number of ways including baking, boiling and mashing. Baked potatoes and sweet potatoes are especially easy to prepare by microwaving for 3 to 5 minutes.

- Desserts—Fresh fruits, nuts, seeds, sugar free ice cream or cakes and pies prepared with sugar substitutes like Stevia.

- Water, milk, yogurt, vegetable juice. Avoid coffee or tea near bedtime. Avoid sweetened colas and alcohol.

- Supplements—Dinner is also a good time to take food supplements.

LUKE CURTIS, MD

Snack Ideas

- Fresh Vegetables such as carrot sticks, celery sticks, broccoli, cherry tomatoes

- Fresh Fruits. Grapes, berries, apples, pears, oranges and bananas are especially popular.

- Popcorn. Popcorn is a whole grain loaded with fiber which makes a wholesome snack. Avoid popcorn candy prepared with large amounts of refined sugar.

- Nuts and Seeds. Peanuts, roasted soybeans, walnuts, cashews, almonds, filberts, Brazil nuts, pecans, sunflower seeds, sesame seeds and pumpkin seeds all make nutritious snack choices. Brazil nuts are especially rich in selenium and the amino acid methionine. Walnuts and pumpkin seeds are rich in valuable omega 3 fats.

- Nut butters such as peanut butter, almond butter and sunflower butter are especially nutritious and are readily available in large supermarkets and health food stores. Look for "natural" peanut butter with no oil on top rather than peanut butter which contains unhealthful hydrogenated vegetable oils.

- Whole grain breads and crackers.

- Milk, yogurt, vegetable juice. Avoid coffee or tea near bedtime.

- Water—Water from the tap is almost free. Flavored water is also available in supermarkets.

- Smoothies—Smoothies can prepared by fruits and vegetables to a base of water or milk. Bananas and blueberries are especially useful to add to smoothies since they provide thickening to the smoothie. Whey protein and other supplements can also be added to smoothies.

Dinning Out Ideas

- Eating out provides a good opportunity to eat new foods and meet new people.

- Eating out provides a good opportunity to try eating seafood such as fish, shellfish, mollusks such as squid, and sea vegetables like kelp. As noted in Chapter 17, many oceanside cultures have enjoyed eating sea animals and vegetables for centuries.

- To save money, many restaurants offer special deals for seniors and/or people who take advantage of other promotions. In many restaurants, lunches are often considerably less expensive than dinners.

- Look for restaurants that provide salad bars. Load up on a wide range of fruits and vegetables and add only a small amounts of dressing. Avoid the croutons, which often contain trans fats.

- Look for restaurants which offer big servings of cooked vegetables. Avoid overcooked vegetables.

- When ordering out sandwiches, always ask that sandwiches be prepared with whole grain breads and with large amounts of vegetables such as tomato, pepper, lettuce, onion and spinach. Subway restaurants offer inexpensive sandwiches made of whole grain bread and many vegetables.

- Water can be ordered to save money in restaurants instead of other drinks.

LUKE CURTIS, MD

Ideas for Elders with Poor Appetites or Digestive Problems

- Drink well balanced nutritional shakes such as Ensure (Abbott) or Boost (Nestle). These nutritional shakes are available in many flavors such as vanilla, chocolate or banana.

- For elders with digestive problems, consider feeding an elemental liquid nutritional formula such as Peptamen AF (Nestle) or Optimental (Abbott). These formulas have predigested protein, fat and carbohydrates. I have seen many severely malnourished elders completely recover after getting these formulas for several weeks. These elders can then go onto to eating food normally

- Consider making or buying high protein smoothies made out of blenderized fruits and vegetables supplemented with whey and/or soy protein. Some commercially available high protein smoothies are available in supermarkets. For example, a 15 ounce Naked Juice's Protein Zone Double Berry Smoothie contains 400 calories, 30 grams protein and 200% of the US RDA for vitamin C.

- Yogurt (from cows or goats milk) is partially digested by the Lactobacillus or Bifidobacterium bacteria and is very easy to digest. Scrambled eggs are also very easy to digest.

- For elders with small appetites, emphasize high protein, high calorie foods like meat, salmon and other fatty fish, cheese, seeds, nuts, peanut butter and other nut butters. Many health food stores have a wide range of delicious nuts and nut butters.

- Digestive enzymes are often helpful for elders with malabsorption problems. Digestive enzymes are available at pharmacies and health food stores.

REFERENCES

1. INTRODUCTION: SENIORS ARE A GROWING AND VITAL PART OF THE POPULATION WHOSE QUALITY OF LIFE IS OFTEN IMPAIRED BY NUTRITIONAL PROBLEMS

ABC News. February 28, 2002. Who goes to church? Older Southern women do; many Catholic men don't. http://abcnews.go.com/sections/us/DailyNews/church_poll020301.html.

AARP (American Association of Retired Persons). 2009. When grandparents provide childcare. http://www.aarp.org/families/grandparents/childcare/when_grandparents_provide_childcare.html.

American Demographics. August 1, 2001. The new family vacation: Demographics, United States. http://findarticles.com/p/articles/mi_m4021/is_2001_August_1/ai_78426765/.

AQHRQ (Agency for Healthcare Research and Quality, USA). Physical activity and older adults. 2000. http://www.ahrq.gov/ppip/activity.htm.

BBC News. April 24, 2007. What are my chances of living to 100?

Beckman, N., M. Waern, D. Gustafson, and I. Skoog. 2008. Secular trends in self-reported sexual activity and satisfaction in Swedish 70 year olds: Cross sectional survey of four populations, 1971-2001. *British Medical Journal* (BMJ) 337:a279.

Bialik, C. April 10, 2008. Hallmark's census of centenarians. Wall Street Journal Blogs.

Congress.org. 2009. Demographics on the 110 Congress. https://ssl.capwiz.com/congressorg/directory/demographics.tt?catid=all.

Hendricks, C. August 17, 2009. Couple maintains world record for longest marriage. *AARP Bulletin*. http://bulletin.aarp.org/yourworld/family/articles/couple_maintains_world_record_for_longest_marriage.html.

Jayson, S. June 2, 2008. Singles find love, marriage after age 45. *USA Today*. http://www.usatoday.com/news/health/2008-06-01-late-life-marriage_N.htm.

Lindau, S. T., L. P. Schumm, E. O. Laumann, W. Levinson, C. O'Muircheartaigh, and L. Waite. 2007. A study of sexuality and health among older adults in the United States. *New England Journal of Medicine* 357(8):762-4.

Messinger-Rapport, B. 2003. Assessment and counseling of older drives: A guide for the primary care physician. *Geriatrics* 58:16-24.

NCSL (National Conference of State Legislatures). 2009. Legislator demographics. http://www.ncsl.org/?tabid=14850.

Society of Actuaries 2000 Mortality Table.

LUKE CURTIS, MD

Superstudy. 1999. Walking is number one. http://walking.about.com/library/weekly/aa081500b.htm.

US Bureau of Labor Statistics. July 2008. Older workers. http://www.bls.gov/spotlight/2008/older_workers/.

US Census. 1996. Nearly 9 in 10 people may marry, but half of all marriages may end in divorce, Census Bureau says. http://www.tia.org/index.html.

US Census. 2001. The 65 and older population. http://www.census.gov/prod/2001pubs/c2kbr01-10.pdf.

US Census Bureau. 2008. International database. Table 094. Midyear population, by age and sex. http://www.census.gov/population/www/projections/natdet-D1A.html.

US Census. 2009. Voting and registration, November 2008 general election. http://www.census.gov/hhes/www/socdemo/voting/index.html.

US Department of Agriculture. 2008. Farm household economics and well-being: Beginning farmers, demographics and labor allocations. http://www.ers.usda.gov/briefing/wellbeing/demographics.htm.

US Travel Industry Association. 1999. Data on trips taken in 1999. http://www.tia.org/index.html.

Webpersonalsonline.com dating demographics 2009. http://www.webpersonalsonline.com/demographics_online_dating.html.

2. MOST OLDER ADULTS ARE MALNOURISHED, WHY?

Adams, K. M., K. C. Lindell, M. Kohlmeier, and S. H. Ziesel. 2006. Status of nutritional education in medical schools. *American Journal of Clinical Nutrition* 83(4):941S-944S.

Andres, E., S. Affenberger, S. Vinzio, et al. 2005. Food-cobalamin malabsorbtion in elderly patients: Clinical manifestations and treatment. *American Journal of Medicine* 118:1154-9.

Auerhahn, C. 1992. Recognition and management of alcohol-related nutritional deficiencies. *Nurse Practitioner* 17(12):40-4.

Bobcock, M. A., and H. H. Keller. 2009. Hospital diagnosis of malnutrition: A call to action. *Canadian Journal of Dietary Practice and Research* 70:37-41.

Brown, T., A. Avenell, L. D. Edmunds, et al. 2009. Systematic review of long-term lifestyle interventions to prevent weight gain and morbidity in adults. *Obesity Reviews* 10:627-38.

Byers, T., M. Nestle, A. McTiernan, C. Doyle, A. Currie-Williams, T. Gansler, and M. Thun. 2002. American Cancer Society guidelines on nutrition and physical activity for cancer prevention. *CA: A Cancer Journal for Clinicians* 52:92-119.

Campbell, I. T. 1999. Limitations of nutrient intake. The effect of stressors: Trauma, sepsis, and multiple organ failure. *European Journal of Clinical Nutrition* 53 Supplement:S143-7.

Crane, S. J., and N. J. Talley. 2007. Chronic gastrointestinal symptoms in the elderly. *Clinics in Geriatric Medicine* 23:721-34.

LUKE CURTIS, MD

Crook, W. 1986. *The yeast connection handbook.* Jackson, Tennessee: Professional Books.

Deruelle, F., and B. Baron. 2008. Vitamin C: Is supplementation necessary for optimal health? *Journal of Alternative and Complimentary Medicine* 14(10):1291-8.

Douglass, C. W., A. Shih, and L. Ostry. 2002. Will there be a need for complete dentures in the United States in 2020? *Journal of Prosthetic Dentistry* 82:5-8.

eMed Expert. 2009. Drugs that cause anorexia as a side effect. http://www.emedexpert.com/side-effects/anorexia.shtml.

Fearon, K. C. H. 2008. Cancer cachexia: Developing a multimodal therapy for multidimensional problems. *European Journal of Cancer* 44:1124-32.

Ginde, A. A., M. C. Liu, C. A. Carlos, et al. 2009. Demographic differences and trends of vitamin D insufficiency in the US population. *Archives of Internal Medicine* 169(9):626-32.

Gorelik, O., D. Almoznion-Sarafian, I. Feder, et al. 2003. Dietary intake of various nutrients in older patients with congestive heart failure. *Cardiology* 99:177-181.

Humbert, I. A., and J. A. Robbins. 2008. Dysphagia in the elderly. *Physical Medicine and Rehabilitation Clinics of North America* 19:853-66.

Inagami, S., D.A. Cohen, A. F. Brown, and S. M. Asch. 2009. Body mass index, neighborhood fast-food and restaurant concentration, and car ownership. *Journal of Urban Health* 86(5):683-95.

Johnson, K. A., M. A. Bernard, and K. Funderberg. 2002. Vitamin nutrition in older adults. *Clinical and Geriatric Medicine* 18:773-99.

Kubrak, C., and L. Jensen. Malnutrition in acute care patients: A narrative review. *International Journal of Nursing Studies* 44:1036-1054.

Lindenbaum, J., I. Rosenberg, P. Wilson, S. Stabler, and R. H. Allen. 1994. Prevalence of cobalmin deficiency in the Framingham elderly population. *American Journal of Clinical Nutrition* 60:2-11.

Linnebur, S. A., S. F. Vondracek, J. P. Vande Griend, J. M. Ruscom, and M. T. McDermott. 2007. Prevalence of vitamin D deficiency in elderly ambulatory patients in Denver, Colorado. *American Journal of Geriatric Pharmacotherapy* 5(1):1-8.

Mancino, L., and J. Buzby. April 2005. Americans' whole grain consumption below guidelines. Amber waves: The economics of food, farming, natural resources and rural America. United States Department of Agriculture. http://www.ers.usda.gov/Amberwaves/April05/Findings/WholeGrainConsumption.htm.

Merck Manual of Geriatrics. 2006. Protein energy undernutrition. http://www.merckmedicus.com/pp/us/hcp/framemm.isp?pg=www.merck.com/pubs/manual/

Meyer, B. J., N. J. Mann, J. L. Lewis, et al. 2003. Dietary intakes and food sources of omega-6 and omega-3 polyunsaturated fatty acids. *Lipids* 38(4):391-8.

Minnesota Board of Aging. 2002. How are older Minnesoatans using prescription drugs? http://www.mnaging.org/advisor/survey/issueBriefs/2002%20IssueBrief-Prescription%20Drug.pdf.

LUKE CURTIS, MD

Morley, J. E., and K. E. Steinberg. 2009. Diarrhea in long-term care: A messy problem. *Journal of the American Medical Directors Association* 10(4):213-7.

Mortality and Morbidity Weekly Reports (MMWR). March 16, 2007. Fruit and vegetable consumption among adults: United States, 2005. MMWR 56(10):213-7. http://www.cdc.gov/mmwr/preview/mmwrhtml/mm5610a2.htm.

Murphy, C. 2008. The chemical senses and nutrition in later years. *Journal of Nutrition for Elders* 27(3-4):247-65.

Nelson, K., M. E. Brown, and N. Lurie. 1998. Hunger in an adult outpatient population. *JAMA (Journal of the American Medical Association)* 279(15):1211-4.

Park, S., M. A. Johnson, and J. G. Fischer. 2008. Vitamin and mineral supplements: Barriers and challenges for older adults. *Journal of Nutrition for the Elderly* 27(3/4):297-317.

Pelton, R. 2009. Drugs that cause nutritional deficiency. http://www.virginiahopkinstestkits.com/nutrientdepl.html.

Prasad, A. S., J. T. Fitzgerald, J. W. Hess, et al. 1993. Zinc deficiency in elderly patients. *Nutrition* 9(3):218-24.

Price, D. M. 2008. Protein-calorie malnutrition in the elderly: implications for nursing care. *Holistic Nursing Practice* 22(6):355-360.

Quandt, S. A., J. MacDonald, T. A. Arcury, et al. 2000. Nutritional self-management of elderly widows in rural communities. *Gerontologist* 40(1):85-6.

Rigler, S. K. 2000. Alcoholism in the elderly. *American Family Physician* 61(6):1883-7.

Rude, R. K., F. R. Singer, and H. E. Gruber. Skeletal and hormonal effects of magnesium deficiency. *Journal of the American College of Nutrition* 28(2):131-41.

Schols, J. M., G. P. De Groot, T. J. Van Der Cammen, and M. G. Olde Rikkert. 2009. Preventing and treating dehydration in the elderly during periods of illness and warm weather. *Journal of Nutrition in Health and Aging* 13(2):150-7.

Sharkey, J. R. 2008. Diet and health outcomes in vulnerable populations. *Annals of the New York Academy of Science* 1136:210-7.

Stechschulte, B. A., R. S. Kirsner, and D. G. Federman. 2009. Vitamin D: Bone and beyond, rationale and recommendation for supplementation. *American Journal of Medicine* 122:793-802.

Stookey, J. D., C. F. Pieper, and H. J. Cohen. 2005. Is the prevalence of dehydration among community-dwelling older adults really low? Informing current debate on the fluid recommendations of adults 70 years or older. *Public Health Nursing* 8(8):1275-85.

Sullivan, R. J. 2005. Fluid intake and hydration: Critical indicators of nursing home quality. *North Carolina Medical Journal* 66(4):296-9.

Schulz, R., S. R. Beach, B. Lind, et al. 2001. Involvement of caregiving and adjustment to death of a spouse: Findings from the caregiver health effects study. *Journal of the American Medical Association* 285(24):3123-9.

Smith, K. L., and C. E. Greenwood. 2008. Weight loss and nutritional considerations in Alzheimer's disease. *Journal of Nutrition for the Elderly* 27(3-4):381-403.

Song, W., O. K. Chun, S. Obayashi, S. Cho, and C. E. Chun. 2005. Is consumption of breakfast associated with body mass index in US adults? *Journal of the American Dietetic Association* 105:1373-82.

Taylor, C. A., J. S. Hampl, and C. S. Johnston. 2000. Low intakes of vegetables and fruits, especially citrus fruits, lead to inadequate vitamin C intakes among adults. *European Journal of Clinical Nutrition* 54:573-8.

Thompson, F. E., T. S. McNeel, E. C. Dowling, et al. 2009. Interrelationships of added sugars intake, socioeconomic status, and race/ethnicity in adults in the United States: National Health Interview Survey, 2005. *Journal of the American Dietetic Association* 109:1376-83.

Timlin, M. T., and M. A. Pereira. 2007. Breakfast frequency and quality in the etiology of adult obesity and chronic diseases. *Nutrition Reviews* (1):268-81.

University of Maryland Medical Center. Drugs that deplete: Coenzyme Q10. http://www.umm.edu/altmed/articles/coenzyme-q10-000706.htm.

US Administration on Aging. 2008. Key indicators of well-being: Health status. http://www.agingstats.gov/agingstatsdotnet/Main_Site/Data/2008_Documents/Highlights.aspx.

United States Department of Health and Human Services. 2000. Healthy people, 2010. Washington, EDC, US Department of Health and Human Services. http://ww.health.gov/healthypeople.

Van Cutsem, E, and J. Arends. 2005. The causes and consequences of cancer-associated malnutrition. *European Journal of Oncology Nursing* 9:S51-S63.

Vaquero, M. P. 2002. Magnesium and trace elements in the elderly: Intake, status, and recommendations. *Journal of Nutrition, Health, and Aging* 6(2):147-53.

Whitney, E., and S. R. Rolfes. 2008. *Understanding nutrition.* Belmont, California: Thompson Wadsworth Publishing.

Wintergerst, E. S., R. Maggini, and D. H. Hornig. 2007. Contribution of selected vitamins and trace elements to immune function. *Annals of Nutrition and Metabolism* 51:301-323.

Wolters, M., A. Strohle, and A. Hahn. 2004. Cobalamin: A critical vitamin in the elderly. *Preventive Medicine* 39(6):1256-66.

3. WEIGHT CONCERNS: IN SENIORS, OVERWEIGHT IS SOMETIMES A PROBLEM, BUT UNDERWEIGHT A MORE COMMON AND OFTENTIMES A WORSE PROBLEM

Agatston, A. 2003. *The South Beach Diet: The delicious, doctor-designed, foolproof plan for fast and healthy weight loss.* New York: St. Martin's Press.

Asomaning, O. L., E. R. Bertone-Johnson, P. C. Nasca, F. Hooven, and P. S. Pekow. 2006. The association between body mass index and osteoporosis in patients referred for a bone mineral density examination. *Journal of Women's Health* 15(9):1028-34.

LUKE CURTIS, MD

Berke, E. M., and N. E. Morden. 2000. Medical management of obesity. *American Family Physician* 62(2):419-26.

Centers for Disease Control. 2009. Overweight and obesity trends among adults. www.cdc.nccdphp/dnpa/obesity/trend/maps/index.htm.

Center on an Aging Society. 2009. Obesity among older Americans. http://www.cdc.gov/nchs/data/databriefs/db01.pdf.

Cloutier, M., and A. Adamson. 2004. The Mediterranean Diet. New York City: Avon Books.

Corrada, M. M., C. H. Kawas, F. Moazaffar, and A. Paganini-Hill. 2006. Association of body mass index and weight change with all-cause mortality in the elderly. *American Journal of Epidemiology* 163:938-949.

Dewys, W., C. Begg, P. Lavin, et al. 1980. Prognostic effect of weight loss prior to chemotherapy in cancer patients. *American Journal of Medicine* 69: 491-497.

He, K., F. B. Hu, G. A. Colditz, et al. 2004. Changes in intake of fruits and vegetables in relation to risk of obesity and weight gain among middle-aged women. *International Journal of Obesity and Related Metabolic Disorders* 28(12):1569-74.

Jannsen, I., and A. E. Mark. 2007. Elevated body mass index and mortality risk in the elderly. *Obesity Research* 8(1):41-59.

Lee, J. S., T. W. Auyeung, T. Kwok, and et al. 2007. Associated factors and health impact of osteoporosis in older Chinese men and women: A cross-sectional study. *Gerontology* 53(6):404-10.

Leon-Munoz, L. M., P. Guallar-Castillion, J. L. Gutierez-Fiasc, et al. 2005. Changes in body weight and health-related quality of life in the older adult population. *International Journal of Obesity* 29(11):1385-91.

McDonald's USA Nutrition Facts for Popular Menu Items. 2009. http://nutrition.mcdonalds.com/nutritionexchange/nutrition_facts. html.

McTigue, K. M., R. Hess, and J. Ziouras J. 2006. Obesity in older adults: A systemic review of the evidence for diagnosis and treatment. *Obesity* 14(9):1485-97.

Raynor, H. A., R. W. Jeffery, A. M. Ruggiero, et al. 2008. Weight loss strategies associated with BMI in overweight adults with type 2 diabetes. *Diabetes Care* 31(7):1299-304.

Sergi, G., E. Perissinotto, C. Pisent, et al. 2005. An adequate threshold for body mass index to detect underweight condition in elderly persons: The Italian Longitudinal Study on Aging (ILSA). *Journal of Gerontology* 60A:7:866-71.

Schneider, S. M., P. Veyres, X. Pivot, et al. 2004. Malnutrition is an independent risk factor associated with nosocomial infections. *British Journal of Nutrition* 92:105-11.

Singh, R. B., V. Rastogi, S. S. Rastogi, et al. 1996. Effect of diet and moderate exercise on central obesity and associated disturbances, myocardial infarction, and mortality in patients with and without coronary artery disease. *Journal of the American College of Nutrition* 15(6):592-601.

LUKE CURTIS, MD

Statistics Canada, Canadian Community Health Survey. 2003. http://www.statcan.gc.ca/pub/82-221-x/2005002/t/html/4150519-eng.htm.

Thalacker-Mercer, A. E., C. A. Johnson, K. E. Yarasheski, N. S. Carnell, and W. W. Campbell. 2007. Nutrient ingestion, protein intake, and sex, but not age, affect the albumin synthesis rate in humans. *Journal of Nutrition* 137:1734-40.

US Department of Agriculture. 2007. Dietary assessment of major trends in US. Food consumption, 1970-2005 by Hodan Wells and Jean Busby. http://www.ers.usda.gov/Publications/EIB33/EIB33.pdf.

WebMD. 2009. Obesity: Health benefits of weight loss. http://www.webmd.com/diet/tc/obesity-health-benefits-of-weight-loss.

4. NUTRITION AND EXERCISE FOR TREATING MUSCLE LOSS (SARCOPENIA)

Baumgartner, R. N., K. M. Koehler, D. Gallagher, et al. 1998. Epidemiology of sarcopenia among the elderly in New Mexico. *American Journal of Epidemiology* 147(8):755-63.

Bischoff-Ferrari, H. A., B. Dawson-Hughes, W. C. Willett, et al. 2004. Effect of vitamin D on falls: A meta-analysis. *Journal of the American Medical Association* 291:1999-2006.

Cosqueric, G., A. Sebag, C. Ducolombier, et al. 2006. Sarcopenia is predictive of nosocomial infection in the elderly. *British Journal of Nutrition* 96: 895-901.

Cawthon, P. M., L. M. Marshall, Y. Michael, et al. 2007. Frailty in older men: Prevalence, progression and relationship with mortality. *Journal of the American Geriatric Society* 55:1216-23.

Clark, R., G. Feleke, M. Din, et al. 2000. Nutritional treatment for acquired immunodeficiency virus-associated wasting using HMB, glutamine and arginine: A double-blind, placebo controlled study. *JPEN* (*Journal of Parenteral and Enteral Nutrition*) 24:133-9.

Fiatarone, M. A., E. C. Marks, N. C. Ryan, et al. 1990. High-intensity strength training in nonagenerians. *Journal of the American Medical Association* 263:3029-34.

Hayes, A., and P. J. Cribb. 2008. Effect of whey protein isolate on strength, body composition and muscle hypertrophy during resistance training. *Current Opinion in Clinical Nutrition and Metabolic Care* 11(1):40-4.

Hughes, V. A., W. R. Frontera, R. Roubenoff, W. J. Evans, and M. A. F. Singh. 2002. Longitudinal changes in body composition in older men and women: Role of body weight change and physical activity. *American Journal of Clinical Nutrition* 76:473-81.

Melov, S., M. A. Tarnopolsky, K. Beckman, K. Felkey, and A. 2007. Hubbard. Resistance exercise reverses aging in human skeletal muscle. *PLoS ONE* 2(5):e465. http://www.plosone.org/article/info:doi%2F10.1371%2Fjournal.pone.0000465.

Jannsen, I., R. N. Baumgartner, R. Ross, I. H. Rosenberg, and R. Roubenoff. 2004. Skeletal muscle cutpoints associated with elevated physical disability risk in older men and women. *American Journal of Epidemiology* 159(4):413-21.

LUKE CURTIS, MD

Kim, J. S., J. M. Wilson, and S. R. Lee. 2010. Dietary implications on mechanisms of sarcopenia: Roles of protein, amino acids and antioxidants. *Journal of Nutritional Biochemistry* In Press.

Siddiqui, R., D. Pandya, K. Harvey, and G. P. Zaloga. 2006. Nutrition modification of cachexia/proteolysis. *Nutrition in Clinical Practice* 21:155-67.

Semba, R. D., F. Lauretani, and L. Ferrucci. 2007. Carotenoids as protection against sarcopenia in older adults. *Archives of Biochemistry and Biophysics* 458:141-145.

Paddon-Jones, D., and B. B. Rasmussen. 2009. Dietary protein recommendations and the prevention of sarcopenia. *Current Opinion in Clinical Nutrition and Metabolic Care* 12:86-90.

Taaffe, D. E. 2006. Sarcopenia: Exercise as a treatment strategy. *Australian Family Physician* 35(3):130-3.

Thomas, D. R. 2007. Loss of lean muscle mass in aging: Examining the relationship of starvation, sarcopenia and cachexia. *Clinical Nutrition* 26: 389-399.

Vaitkevincius, P. V., C. Ebersold, M. S. Shah, et al. 2002. Effects of exercise training in community-based subjects aged 80 and older: A pilot study. *Journal of the American Geriatric Society* 59:2009-13.

Zacker, R. J. 2006. Health-related implications and management of sarcopenia. *Journal of the American Association of Physician Assistants* 19(10):24-9.

Zamboni, M., G. Mazzali, F. Fantin, A. Rossi, and V. Di Francesco V. 2008. Sarcopenia obesity: A new category of obesity in the elderly. *Nutrition, Metabolism and Cardiovascular Disease* 18(5):388-95.

5. NUTRITION AND EXERCISE FOR TREATING BONE LOSS (OSTEOPOROSIS)

Bischoff-Ferrari, H. A., W. C. Willet, J. B. Wong, et al. 2009. Prevention of non-vertebral fractures with oral vitamin D and dose dependency. *Archives of Internal Medicine* 169(6):551-61.

Braam, L. A., M. H. Knapen, P. Gueusens, et al. 2003. Vitamin K supplementation retards bone loss in postmenopausal women between ages of 50 and 60 years. *Calciferous Tissue International* 73(1):21-6.

Dimal, H. P., S. Porta, G. Wirnsberger, et al. 1998. Daily oral magnesium supplementation suppresses bone turnover in the young male. *Journal of Clinical Endocrinology and Metabolism* 83(8):2742-8.

Guadalupe-Grau, A., T. Fuentes, B. Guerra, and J. A. L. Calbet. 2009. Exercise and bone mass in adults. *Sports Medicine* 39(6):439-468.

Hooshmand, S., and B. H. Arjmandi. 2009. Viewpoint: Dried plum, an emerging functional food that may effectively improve bone health. *Ageing Research Reviews* 8:122-7.

Ishimi, Y. 2009. Soybean isoflavones in bone health. *Forums in Nutrition* 61:104-16.

Kamel, H. K. 2006. Postmenopausal osteoporosis: Etiology, current diagnostic strategies and non-prescriptions interventions. *Journal of Managed Care Pharmacy* 12:S4-9.

LUKE CURTIS, MD

Kanis, J., H. Johansson, A. Oden, et al. 2006. A meta-analysis of milk intake and fracture risk: Low utility and case finding. *Osteoporosis International* 16:799-804.

Kitchin, B., and S. L. Morgan. 2007. Not just calcium and vitamin D: Other nutritional considerations in osteoporosis. *Current Rheumatology Reports* 9:85-92.

Kruger, M. C., H. Coetzer, R. De Winter, G. Gericke, and D. H. Van Papendorp. Calcium, gamma-linolenic acid and eicosapentaenoic acid supplementation in senile osteoporosis. *Aging (Milano)* 10(5):385-94.

Meunier, P. J., C. Roux, E. Seeman, et al. 2004. The effects of strontium ranelate on the risk of vertebral fracture in women with postmenopausal osteoporosis. *New England Journal of Medicine* 350:5:459-68.

Morton, D., E. Barrett-Conner, and D. L. Schneider. 2001. Vitamin C supplement use and bone mineral density in postmenopausal women. *Journal of Bone and Mineral Research* 16:135-40.

Palacios, C. 2006. The role of nutrients in bone health from A to Z. *Critical Reviews in Food Science and Nutrition* 46:621-8.

Park, S., M. A. Johnson, and J. G. Fischer. 2008. Vitamin and mineral supplements: Barriers and challenges for older adults. *Journal of Nutrition for the Elderly* 27(3/4):297-317.

Rude, R. K., F. R. Singer, and H. E. Gruber. 2009. Skeletal and hormonal effects of magnesium deficiency. *Journal of the American College of Nutrition* 28(2):131-41.

Sahni, S., M. T. Hannan, D. Gagnon, et al. 2009. Protective effect of total and supplemental vitamin C intake on the risk of hip fracture: A 17-year follow-up from the Framingham Osteoporosis Study. *Osteoporosis International* 20(11):1853-61.

Sahni, S., M. T. Hannan, J. Blumberg, et al. 2009. Protective effect of total carotenoid and lycopene intake on the risk of hip fracture: A 17-year follow-up from the Framingham Osteoporosis Study. *Journal of Bone and Mineral Research* 24:1086-94.

Seeman, E., S. Boonen, S. Boergstrom, et al. 2009. Five years treatment with strontium ranelate reduces vertebral and nonvertebral fractures and increases the number of quality of remaining life years in women over 80 years of age. *Bone* In Press.

Stechschulte, B. A., R. S. Kirsner, and D. G. Federman. 2009. Vitamin D: Bone and beyond, rationale and recommendation for supplementation. *American Journal of Medicine* 122:793-802.

Sweet, M. G., J. M. Sweet, M. P. Jeremiah, and S. S. Galazka. 2009. Diagnosis and treatment of osteoporosis. *American Family Physician* 79(3):193-200.

Tang, B., G. Eslick, C. Nolwson, et al. 2007. Use of calcium in combination with vitamin D supplementation to prevent fractures and bone loss in people aged 50 years and older: A meta-analysis. *Lancet* 370:657-66.

Walker, M., P. Klentrou, R. Chow, and M. Plyley. 2000. Longitudinal evaluation of supervised versus unsupervised exercise programs for the treatment of osteoporosis. *European Journal of Applied Physiology* 83:349-355.

LUKE CURTIS, MD

Vanderput, L., and C. Ohksson. 2009. Estrogens as regulators of bone health in men. *Nature Review in Endocrinology* 5(8):437-443.

Whitney, E., and S. R. Rolfes. 2008. *Understanding nutrition.* Belmont, California: Thompson Wadsworth Publishing.

Yaegashi, Y., T. Onoda, K. Tanno, T. Kuribayashi, K. Sakata, and H. Orimo. 2008. Association of hip fracture incidence and intake of calcium, magnesium, vitamin D, and vitamin K. *European Journal of Epidemiology* 23:219-225.

6. NUTRITION TO PREVENT AND TREAT INFECTION

Aul, C., U. Germing, N. Gatterman, and H. Minning. 1998. Increased incidence of myelodysplastic syndromes: Real or fictitious? *Leukemia Research* 22(1):93-100.

Avenell, A., J. A. Cook, G. S. MacLennan, and G. C. MacPherson. 2007. Vitamin D supplementation to prevent infections: A sub-study of a randomized placebo-controlled trial in older people. *Age and Ageing* 36:574-92.

Caulfield, L. E., M. De Orris, M. Blossner, and R. F. Black. 2004. Undernutrition as an underlying cause of child deaths associated with diarrhea, pneumonia, malaria and measles. *American Journal of Clinical Nutrition* 80:193-8.

CIDRAP. 2008. Death rate for flu, pneumonia fell sharply in 2006. http://www.cidrap.umn.edu/cidrap/content/influenza/general/news/jun1208deaths-br.html.

Curtis, L. 2008. Nutrition, copper and myelodysplasia. *Transfusion Medicine* 18:315-6.

_____. 2008. Prevention of hospital-acquired infections: Review of non-pharmacological interventions. *Journal of Hospital Infection* 69:204-219.

Douglas, R. M., H. Hemila, E. Chalker, and B. Treacy. July 18, 2007. Vitamin C in preventing and treating the common cold. *Cochrane Database System Review* CD000980.

Foxman, B. 2002. Epidemiology of urinary tract infections: Incidence, morbidity and economic costs. *American Journal of Medicine* 113(1A):5S-13S.

Fujisawa, H., K. Watanabe, K. Suma, et al. 2009. Antibacterial potential of garlic-derived allicin and its canellation by sulfhydryl compounds. *Bioscience, Biotechnology and Biochemistry* 73(9):1948-55.

Guinan, M., M. McGuckin, and Y. Ali. 2002. The effect of a comprehensive handwashing program on absenteeism in elementary schools. *American Journal of Infection Control* 30:217-20.

Jackson, J. L., E. Lesho, and C. Peterson. 2000. Zinc and the common cold: Meta-analysis revisited. *Journal of Nutrition* 130(5 Supplement):12S-5S.

Jepson, R., and J. C. Craig. 2007. A systematic review of the evidence for cranberries and blueberries in UTI prevention. *Molecular Nutrition and Food Research* 51:738-45.

Johansson, N. L., C. S. Pavia, and J. W. Chiao. 2008. Growth inhibition for a spectrum of bacterial and fungal pathogens by sulforaphane, an isocyanate product found in broccoli and other cruciferous vegetables. *Planta Medica* 74(7):747-50.

LUKE CURTIS, MD

Li, L., and M. M. Werler. 2009. Fruit and vegetable intake and risk of upper respiratory tract infection in pregnant women. *Public Health Nutrition* In Press.

Liu, B. S., A. McGeer, M. A. McArthur, et al. 2007. Effect of a multivitamin and mineral supplement on episodes of infection in nursing home residents: A randomized, placebo-controlled study. *Journal of the American Geriatric Society* 55(1):35-42.

McMurdo, M. E. T., I. Argo, G. Phillips, et al. 2009. Cranberry or trimethoprim for the prevention of recurrent urinary tract infections? A randomized controlled trial in older women. *Journal of Antimicrobial Chemotherapy* 63:389-95.

Merchant, A. T., G. C. Curhan, E. B. Rimm, et al. 2005. Intake of omega-6 and omega-3 fatty acids and risk of community acquired pneumonia in US men. *American Journal of Clinical Nutrition* 82(3):668-74.

NIAID. 2001. The common cold, NIAID fact sheet. http://www.wrongdiagnosis.com/artic/the_common_cold_niaid_fact_sheet_niaid.htm.

Paillaud, E., S. Herbaud, P. Caillet, et al. 2005. Relations between undernutrition and nosocomial infection in elderly patients. *Age and Ageing* 34:619-25.

Reid, G., and A. W. Bruce. 2006. Probiotics to prevent urinary tract infections: The rationale and evidence. *World Journal of Urology* 24:28-32.

Rothan-Tondeur, M., S. Meaume, L. Girard, et al. 2003. Risk factors for nosocomial pneumonia in a geriatric hospital: A case-control, one-center study. *Journal of the American Geriatric Society* 51(7):997-1001.

Roxas, M., and J. Jurenka. 2007. Colds and influenza: a review of diagnosis and conventional, botanical and nutritional considerations. *Alternative Medicine Review* 12(1):25-48.

Schneider, S. M., P. Veyres, X. Pivot, et al. 2004. Malnutrition is an independent risk factor associated with nosocomial infections. *British Journal of Nutrition* 92:105-11.

Shah, S. A., S. Sander, C. M. White, et al. 2007. Evaluation of Echinacea for the prevention and treatment of the common cold: A meta-analysis. *Lancet Infectious Diseases* 7(7):473-80.

Simoes, M., R. N. Bennett, and E. A. S. Rosa. 2009. Understanding antimicrobial activities of phytochemicals against multidrug resistant bacteria and biofilms. *Natural Products Reports* 26:746-57.

Stephen, A. I., and A. Avenell. 2006. A systematic review of multivitamin and mineral supplementation for infection. *Journal of Human Nutrition and Dietetics* 19:179-90.

Thomson, C. D., A. Chisholm, S. K. McLachlen, and J. M. Campbell. 2008. Brazil nuts an effective way to improve selenium status. *American Journal of Clinical Nutrition* 87(2):379-84.

Vouloumanou, E. K., G. C. Makris, D. E. Karargeorgopoulous, and M. E. Falagas. 2009. Probiotics for the prevention of respiratory tract infections: A systemic review. *International Journal of Antimicrobial Agents* 34:197e.1-197.e.10.

White, C., R. Kolble, R. Carlson, and N. Lipson. 2005. The impact of a health campaign on hand hygiene and upper respiratory illness among college students living in residence halls. *Journal of American College Health* 53(4):175-81.

Weiner, C., Q. Pan, M. Hurtig, et al. 1999. Passive immunity against human pathogens using bovine antibodies. *Clinical and Experimental Immunology* 116:193-205.

Wintergerst, E. S., R. Maggini, and D. H. Hornig. 2007. Contribution of selected vitamins and trace elements to immune function. *Annals of Nutrition and Metabolism* 51:301-23.

Yalcin, A. S. 2006. Emerging therapeutic potential of whey proteins and peptides. *Current Pharmaceutical Design* 12:1637-43.

7. BETTER HOSPITAL NUTRITION IS CRITICAL FOR RECOVERY

Adams, K. M., K. C. Lindell, M. Kohlmeier, and S. H. Ziesel. 2006. Status of nutritional education in medical schools. *American Journal of Clinical Nutrition* 83(4):941S-944S.

Andel, H., L. P. Kamolz, K. Horauf, and M. Zimpfer. 2003. Nutrition and anabolic agents in burned patients. *Burns* 29:592-5.

Beale, R. J., R. Sherry, K. Lei, et al. 2008. Early enteral supplementation with key phamaconutrients improves Sequential Organ Failure Assessment score in critically ill patients with sepsis: Outcome of a randomized, controlled, double-blind study. *Critical Care Med.* 36(1):131-44.

Bobcock, M. A., and H. H. Keller. 2009. Hospital diagnosis of malnutrition: A call to action. *Canadian Journal of Dietary Practice and Research* 70:37-41.

Centers for Disease Control. 2006. Fire deaths and injuries: Fact sheet. http://www.cdc.gov/HomeandRecreationalSafety/Fire-Prevention/fires-factsheet.htmlt.

Curtis, L. 2002. Burning Issues: Wood, forests, grass, leaf and trash burning. *Human Ecologist*, Fall 95:25-29.

_____. 2008. Prevention of hospital-acquired infections: Review of non-pharmacological interventions. *Journal of Hospital Infection* 69:204-19.

DeLegge, M. H. 2008. Enteral feeding. *Current Opinion in Gastroenterology* 24(2):184-9.

Doig, G. S., P. T. Heighes, F. Simpson, E. A. Sweetman, and A. R. Davies. 2009. Early enteral nutrition, provided within 24 hours of injury or intensive care unit admission, significantly reduces mortality in critically ill patients: A meta-analysis of randomized controlled trials. *Intensive Care Medicine* 35:2018-27.

Fire Safety for Citizens. 2010. Smoking fire safety. http://www.firesafety.gov/citizens/firesafety/smoking.shtm.

Gudaviciene, D., R. Rimdeika, and K. Adamonis. 2004. Nutrition of burned patients. *Medicina* (Kaunas) 40(1):1-8.

Hickson, M., A. L. D'Souza, N. Muthu, et al. 2007. Use of probiotic Lactobacillus preparation to prevent diarrhea associated with antibiotics: Randomised double blind controlled trial. *British Medical Journal* 335:80-4.

Johnson, S., R. Nasser, T. Banow, T. Cockburn, L. Voegeli, O. Wilson, and J. Coleman. 2009. Use of oral nutritional supplements

LUKE CURTIS, MD

in long-term care facilities. *Canadian Journal of Diet Practice and Research* 70(4):194-8.

Kubrak, C., and L. Jensen. 2007. Malnutrition in acute care patients: A narrative review. *International Journal of Nursing Studies* 44:1036-1054.

Manley, K. J., M. B. Fraenkel, B. C. Mayall, and D. A. Power. 2007. Probiotic treatment of vancomycin-resistant enterococci: A randomized controlled trial. *Medical Journal of Australia* 186:454-7.

Marik, P. E., and G. P. Zaloga. 2008. Immunonutrition in critically ill patients: A systemic review and analysis of the literature. *Intensive Care Medicine* 24:1980-90.

Mattei, P., and J. L. Rombeau. 2006. Review of pathophysiology and management of postoperative ileus. *World Journal of Surgery* 30:1382-91.

McFarland, L. 2006. Meta-analysis of probiotics for the prevention of antibiotic associated diarrhea and the treatment of Clostridium difficile disease. *American Journal of Gastroenterol* 101:812-22.

Montejo, J. C., A. Zarazaga, J. Lopez-Martinez, et al. 2003. Immunonutrition in the intensive care unit. A systemic review and consensus statement. *Clinical Nutrition* 22:221-33.

Nightingale, F. 1859. *Notes on Nursing: What it is and what it is not.* London, Great Britain: Hanson and Sons.

Schneider, S. M., P. Veyres, X. Pivot, et al. 2004. Malnutrition is an independent risk factor associated with nosocomial infections. *British Journal of Nutrition* 92:105-11.

Wibbenmeyer, L. A., M. A. Amelon, R. M. Loret-De Mola, et al. 2003. Trash and brush burning: An underappreciated mechanism of thermal injury in a rural community. *Journal of Burn Care and Rehabilitation* 24(2):85-9.

Wintergerst, E. S., R. Maggini, and D. H. Hornig. 2007. Contribution of selected vitamins and trace elements to immune function. *Annals of Nutrition and Metabolism* 51:301-23.

Zippi, M., S. Fiorani, I. De Felici, I. Febbraro, et al. 2009. Percutaneous endoscopic gastromy (PEG) in critically ill patients performed at bed in the Intensive Care Unit: Report of our experience. *Clinical Therapeutics* 160(5):359-62.

8. NUTRITION TO IMPROVE HEART, ARDIOVASCULAR, AND LUNG HEALTH AND PREVENT HEART DISEASE, STROKE, AND ASTHMA

Albert, A., C. Altabre, F. Baro, et al. 202. Efficacy and safety of a phytoestrogen preparation derived from glycine max (L) in climacteric symptomatology. *Phytomedicine* 9:85-92.

Alonso, A., C. DeLaFunete, A. M. Martin-Arnau, et al. 2004. Fruit and vegetable consumption is inversely associated with blood pressure in a Mediterranean population with a high-vegetable-fat intake: The Seguimiento Universidad de Navarra (SUN) study. *British Journal of Nutrition* 92:311-9.

American Heart Association. 2009. Heart disease and stroke statistics. http://www.americanheart.org/downloadable/heart/123 783441267009Heart%20and%20Stroke%20Update.pdf.

LUKE CURTIS, MD

American Heart Association. 2010. What is atherosclerosis? http://www.americanheart.org/presenter.jhtml?identifier=4440.

Andrews, J., J. Heath, L. Harrell, and H. Forbes. 2000. Meeting national tobacco challenges: Recommendations for stop smoking groups. *Journal of the American Academy of Nurse Practitioners* 12(12):522-30.

Ball, K. P., E. Hanington, P. M. McAllen, et al. 1965. Low-fat diet in myocardial infarction: A controlled trial. *Lancet* 2:501-4.

Baldassarre, D., S. Castelnuvio, B. Frigerio, et al. 2009. Effects of timing and extent of smoking types of cigarettes, and concomitant risk factors on the association between smoking and subclinical atherosclerosis. *Stroke* 40(6):1991-8.

Banel, D. K., and F. Hu. 2009. Effects of walnut consumption on blood lipids and other cardiovascular risk factors: A meta-analysis and systematic review. *American Journal of Clinical Nutrition* 90:56-63.

Benavente-Garcia, O., and J. Castillo. 2008. Update on uses of citrus flavonoids: New findings in anticancer, cardiovascular and anti-inflammatory activity. *Journal of Agricultural and Food Chemistry* 56:6185-205.

Berne, R. M., and M. N. Levy. 2008. *Physiology*. 4th ed. St. Louis, Missouri: Mosby.

Berry, J. K., and C. L. Baum. 2001. Malnutrition in chronic obstructive pulmonary disease: Adding insult to injury. *AACN Clinical Issues* 12(2):210-9.

Blanchard, C. M., J. Fisher, P. B. Sparling, et al. 2009. Understanding adherence to 5 to 6 servings a day of fruits and vegetables. *Journal of Nutrition Education and Behavior* 41(1):3-10.

Brown, L., F. Sachs, B. Rosner, and W. C. Willett. 1999. Nut consumption and risk of coronary heart disease in patients with coronary heart disease (Abstract). *FASEB Journal* 13:A4332.

Brown, L., B. Rosner, W. W. Willett, and F. B. Sacks. 1999. Cholesterol-lowering effects of dietary fiber: A meta-analysis. *American Journal of Clinical Nutrition* 69:30-42.

Buil-Cosiales, P., P. Irimia, N. Berrade, et al. 2008. Carotid intima-media thickness is inversely associated with olive oil consumption. *Atherosclerosis* 196:742-8.

Burr, M. L., A. M. Fehily, F. Gilbert, et al. 1989. Effects of changes in fat, fish and fibre intakes on death and myocardial reinfarction. Diet and reinfarction trial (DART). *Lancet* 2:757-61.

Carrero, J. J., and R. F. Grimble. 2006. Does nutrition have a role in peripheral vascular disease? *British Journal of Nutrition* 95(2):217-29.

Caso, G., P. Kelly, M. A. McNurlan, and W. E. Lawson. 2007. Effect of coenzyme Q_{10} on myopathic symptoms in patients treated with statins. *American Journal of Cardiology* 99(10):1409-12.

Cavallini, G., S. Caracciolo, G. Vitali, et al. 2004. Carnitine versus androgen administration in the treatment of sexual dysfunction, depressed mood, and fatigue associated with male aging. *Urology* 63(4):641-6.

LUKE CURTIS, MD

Chen, Z. Y., R. Jiao, and K. Y. Ma. 2008. Cholesterol-lowering nutraceuticals and functional foods. *Journal of Agricultural and Food Chemicals* 56:8761-73.

Chen, Z. Y., C. Peng, R. Jiao, et al. 2009. Anti-hypertensive nutraceuticals and functional foods. *Journal of Agricultural and Food Chemistry* 57:4485-99.

Chen, J., Y. Wollman, T. Chernichovsky, et al. 1999. Effect of oral administration of high-dose nitric oxide donor L-arginine in men with organic erectile dysfunction: Results of a double-blind, randomized, placebo-controlled study. *BJU International* 83:269-73.

Cheuk, D. 2005. A meta-analysis of intravenous magnesium sulphate for treating acute asthma. *Archives of Disease in Childhood* 90(1):74-7.

Curtis, L., W. Rea, P. Smith, and Y. Pan. 2006. Adverse health effects of outdoor air pollution. *Environment International* 32(6):815-30.

Curtis, L, A. Lieberman, W. Rea, M. Stark, and M. Vetter. 2004. Health effects of indoor mold exposure. *Journal of Nutritional and Environmental Medicine* (3):261-74.

Cutler, J. A., P. D. Sorlie, M. Wolz, et al. 2008. Trends in hypertension prevalence, awareness, treatment, and control rates in United States adults between 1988-1994 and 1999-2004. *Hypertension* 58:818-27.

Digby, J. E., J. M. Lee, and R. P. Choudhury. 2009. Nicotinic acid and the prevention of coronary artery disease. *Current Opinion in Lipidology* 20(4):321-6.

Doolan, D. M., and E. S. Froelicher. 2008. Smoking cessation interventions and older adults. *Progress in Cardiovascular Nursing* 23:119-27.

Ellingsen, I., I. Seljeflot, H. Arnesen, and S. Tonstad. 2009. Vitamin C consumption is associated with less regression in carotid intima thickness in elderly men: A 3-year intervention study. *Nutrition, Metabolism and Cardiovascular Disease* 19(1):8-14.

Elwood, P. C., J. J. Strain, P. J. Robson, et al. 2005. Milk consumption, stroke, and heart attack risk: Evidence from the Caerphilly cohort of older men. *Journal of Epidemiology and Community Health* 59(6):502-5.

Erkkila, A. T., A. H. Lichtenstein, D. Mozaffarian, and D. M. Herrington. 2004. Fish intake is associated with a reduced progression of coronary artery atherosclerosis in postmenopausal women with coronary artery disease. *American Journal of Clinical Nutrition* 80(3):626-32.

eMedicine. 2009. High blood pressure. http://www. emedicinehealth.com/high_blood_pressure/article_em.htm.

Eshah, N., and A. E. Bond. 2009. Cardiac rehabilitation programme for coronary heart disease patients: An integrative literature review. *International Journal of Nursing Practice* 15:131-9.

Esposito, K., M. Ciotola, F. Giugluiano, et al. 2006. Mediterranean diet improves erectile function in subjects with the metabolic syndrome. *International Journal of Impotence Research* 18:405-10.

Flores-Mateo, G., A. Navas-Acien, A. Pastor-Barriuso, and E. Guallar. 2006. Selenium and coronary heart disease: A meta-analysis. *American Journal of Clinical Nutrition* 84(4):762-73.

LUKE CURTIS, MD

Fogarty, A., and J. Britton. 2000. The role of diet in the aetiology of asthma. *Clinical and Experimental Allergy* 30:615-27.

Foley, N., R. E. Martin, K. L. Salter, and R. W. Teasell. 2009. A review of the relationship between dysphagia and malnutrition following stroke. *Journal of Rehabilitation Medicine* 41(9):707-13.

Friedman, E., and S. A. Thomas. 1995. Pet ownership, social support, and one-year survival after acute myocardial infarction in the cardiac arrhythmia suppression trial (CAST). *American Journal of Cardiology* 76:1213-7.

Ghandehari, H., S. Kamal-Bahl, and N. D. Wong. 2008. Prevalence and extent of dyslipidemia and recommended lipid levels in US adults with and without cardiovascular comorbidities. *American Heart Journal* 156:112-9.

Glantz, S. A., and W.W. Parmley. 1991. Passive smoking and heart disease: Epidemiology, physiology and biochemistry. *Circulation* 83(1):1-12.

Hall, S. A., R. Shackleton, R. C. Rosen, and A. B. Araujo. 2010. Sexual activity, erectile dysfunction and incident cardiovascular events. *American Journal of Cardiology* 105(2):192-7.

Hanna, I. R., and N. K. Wenger. 2005. Secondary prevention of coronary heart disease in elderly patients. *American Family Physician* 17:2289-96.

Harland, J. I., and T. A. Haffner. 2008. Systematic review, meta-analysis and regression of randomized controlled trials reporting an association between an intake of cica 25 grams soya protein per day and blood cholesterol. *Atherosclerosis* 200(1):13-27.

He, F. J., C. A. Nowson, and G. A. MacGregor. 2006. Fruit and vegetable consumption and stroke: Meta-analysis of cohort studies. *Lancet* 367:320-6.

Heffernan, K. S., C. A. Fahs, S. M. Ranadive, and E. A. Patvardhan. 2010. L-arginine as a nutritional prophylaxis against vascular dysfunction with gaining. *Journal of Cardiovascular Pharmacological Therapies* In Press.

Heron, M., D. Hoyert, S. L. Murophy, et al. 2009. National vital statistics reports: Deaths: Final data for 2006. Volume 15, number 14. http://www.cdc.gov/nchs/data/nvsr/nvsr57/nvsr57_14.pdf.

Hu, F. B., and W. C. Willett. 2002. Optimal diets for prevention of coronary heart disease. *Journal of the American Medical Association* 288:2569-78.

Hua, L., A. Brown, S. Hains, et al. 2009. Effects of low-intensity exercise conditioning on blood pressure, heart rate and autonomic modulation of heart rate in men and women with hypertension. *Biological Research for Nursing* 11(2):129-43.

Hubayter, Z., and J. A. Simon. 2008. Testosterone therapy for sexual dysfunction in postmenopausal women. *Climacteric* 11:181-91.

Ito, T., M. Polan, S. Whipple, and A. S. Trant. 2006. The enhancement of female sexual function with AgrinMax, a nutritional supplement, among women differing in menopausal status. *Journal of Sex and Marital Therapy* 32:369-78.

Jaakkola, M. S. 2002. Environmental tobacco smoke in the elderly. *European Respiratory Journal* 19(1):172-81.

LUKE CURTIS, MD

Jee, S.H., E. R. Miller, E. Guallar, et al. 2006. The effect of magnesium supplementation on blood pressure: A meta-analysis of randomized clinical trials. *American Journal of Hypertension* 15:691-6.

Jeejeebhoy, F., M. Keith, M. Freeman, et al. 2002. Nutritional supplementation with MyoVive repletes essential cardiac myocyte nutrients and reduces left ventricular size in patients with left ventricular dysfunction. *American Heart Journal* 143:1092-100.

Karppanen, H., P. Karppanen, and E. Mervaala. 2005. Why and how to implement sodium, potassium, calcium and magnesium changes in food items and diet. *Journal of Human Hypertension* 19(Supplement 3):S10-9.

Karppanen, H., and E. Mervaala. 2006. Sodium intake and hypertension. *Progress in Cardiovascular Disease* 9:59-75.

Knekt, P., J. Ritz, M. Pereira, et al. 2004. Antioxidant vitamins and coronary heart disease risk: A pooled analysis of 9 cohorts. *American Journal of Clinical Nutrition* 80:1508-20.

Kris-Etherton, P., J. A. Grieger, K. F. Hilpert, and S. G. 2009. West. Milk products, dietary patterns and blood pressure management. *Journal of the American College of Nutrition* 28(Supplement 1):103S-19S.

Kris-Etherton, P., A. H. Lichtenstein, B. V. Howard, et al. 2004. Antioxidant vitamins and cardiovascular disease. *Circulation* 110:637-41.

Lapretre, P. M., T. Vogel, P. H. Brechat, et al. 2009. Impact of short-term aerobic interval training on maximal exercise in sedentary aged subjects. *International Journal of Clinical Practice* 63(10):1472-8.

Lavie, C. J., R. V. Milani, M. R. Mehra, and H. O. Ventura. 2009. Omega-3 polyunsaturated fatty acids and cardiovascular diseases. *Journal of the American College of Cardiology* 54(7):585-94.

Lett, H. S., J. A. Blumenthal, M. A. Babyak, et al. 2005. Social support and coronary heart disease: Epidemiological evidence and implications for treatment. *Psychosomatic Medicine* 869-78.

Likourezos, A., and O. R. Burack. 2002. The therapeutic use of companion animals. *Clinical Geriatrics* 10(4):31-3.

Logemann, J. A. 2007. Swallowing disorders. *Best Practice Research in Clinical Gastroenterology* 21(4):563-73.

Manz, F., and A. Wentz. 2005. The importance of good hydration for the prevention of chronic diseases. *Nutrition Reviews* 63(6 Part 2):S2-S5.

Marchioli, R., C. Scheiger, L. Tavazzi, and F. Valagussa. 2001. Efficacy of n-3 polyunsaturated fatty acids after myocardial infarcation: Results of the GISSI-Prevenzione trial. *Lipids* 36(Supplement):119-26.

Martins, I. J., T. Berger, M. J. Sharman, et al. 2009. Cholesterol metabolism and transport in the pathogenesis of Alzheimer's disease. *Journal of Neurochemistry* 111(6):1275-308.

McKenney, J. M., and D. Sica. 2007. Prescription omega-3 fatty acids for the treatment of hypertriglycerdemia. *American Journal of Health Systems Pharmacy* 64:595-605.

LUKE CURTIS, MD

Meijer, W. T., A. W. Hoes, M. Rutgers, et al. 1998. Peripheral arterial disease in the elderly: The Rotterdam study. *Arteriosclerosis, Thrombosis and Vascular Biology* 18(2):185-92.

Mortality and Morbidity Weekly Reports (MMWR). March 16, 2007. Fruit and vegetable consumption among adults: United States, 2005. *MMWR* 56(10):213-7. http://www.cdc.gov/mmwr/preview/mmwrhtml/mm5610a2.htm.

National Institutes of Health. 2009. Data fact sheet: Asthma statistics. http://www.nhlbi.nih.gov/health/prof/lung/asthma/asthstat.pdf.

Oxman, T. E., D. H. Freeman, and E. D. Manheimer. 1995. Lack of social participation or religious strength and comfort as risk factors for death in cardiac surgery in the elderly. *Psychosomatic Medicine* 57(1):5-15.

Paddock, C. February 25, 2008. Cat owners has lower heart attack risk. *Medical News Today*. http://www.medicalnewstoday.com/articles/98432.php.

Pittler, M. H., and E. Ernst. 2005. Complementary therapies for peripheral arterial disease: Systematic review. *Atherosclerosis* 181:1-7.

Romieu, I., and C. Trenga. 2001. Diet and obstructive lung disease. *Epidemiology Review* 23(2): 268-87.

Sacks, F. M., L. P. Svetkey, W. M. Vollmer, et al. 2001. Effects on blood pressure and reduced dietary sodium and the dietary approaches to stop hypertension (DASH) diet. *New England Journal of Medicine* 334:3-10.

Sanchez-Moreno, C., A. Jimenez-Escrig, and A. Martin. 2009. Stroke: Roles of B vitamins, homocysteine and anti-oxidants. *Nutrition Research Reviews* 22(1):49-67.

Selvin, E., A. Burrnett, and E. A. Platz. 2007. Prevalence and risk factors for erectile dysfunction in the US. *American Journal of Medicine* 120:151-7.

Sharlip, I. D., B. P. Schumaker, L. S. Hakim, et al. 2008. Tadafil is efficacious and well tolerated in the treatment of erectile dysfunction (ED) in men over 65 years of age. *Journal of Sexual Medicine* 5(3):716-25.

Shechter, M., and A. Shechter. 2005. Magnesium and myocardial infarction. *Clinical Calcium* 15(11):111-5.

Shim, C., and H. Williams. 1986. Effect of odors in asthma. *American Journal of Medicine* 80(1):18-22.

Soukoulis, V., B. Dih, M. Sole, et al. 2009. Micronutrient deficiencies: An unmet need in heart failure. *Journal of the American College of Cardiology* 54(18):1660-73.

Spence, J. D. 2006. Nutrition and stroke prevention. *Stroke* 37:2430-5.

Taylor, D. H., V. Hasselblad, J. Henley, et al. 2002. Benefits of smoking cessation for longevity. *American Journal of Public Health* 92(6):990-6.

Taylor, R. S., A. Brown, S. Ebrahim, et al. 2004. Exercise-based rehabilitation for patients with coronary heart disease: Systematic review and meta-analysis of randomized controlled trials. *American Journal of Medicine* 116:682-92.

LUKE CURTIS, MD

Turgut, F., M. Kambay, M. R. Metin, et al. 2008. Magnesium supplementation helps improve carotid intima media thickness in patients on hemodialysis. *International Urology and Nephrology* 40(4):1075-82.

Van Dumme, Y. M., K. M. Verhamme, T. Stijnen, et al. 2009. Prevalence, incidence and lifetime risk for the development of COPD in the elderly: The Rotterdam Study. *Chest* 135(2): 3698-77.

Van Horn, L. V., M. McCoin, P. M. Kris-Etherton, et al. 2008. The evidence for dietary prevention and treatment of cardiovascular disease. *Journal of the American Dietetic Association* 108:287-331.

Van Mierlo, L. A. J., L. R. Arends, and M. T. Streppel. 2006. Blood pressure in relation to calcium supplementation: A meta-analysis of randomized controlled trials. *Journal of Human Hypertension* 20:571-80.

Verissimo, M. T., A. Aragao, A. Sousa, et al. 2002. Effect of physical exercise on lipid metabolism in the elderly. *Reviews of Portuguese Cardiology* 21(10):1099-112.

WebMD. 2009. Cholesterol management guide. http://www.webmd.com/cholesterol-management/guide/diseases-linked-high-cholesterol.

Webpersonalsonline.com dating demographics. 2009. http://www.webpersonalsonline.com/demographics_online_dating.html.

Wildman, R. P., L. L. Schott, S. Brockwell, et al. 2004. A dietary and exercise intervention slows menopause-associated progression of subclinical atherosclerosis as measured by intima-media thickness of the carotid arteries. *Journal of the American College of Cardiology* 44(3):579-85.

Yabroff, K. R., R. P. Troiano, and D. Berrigan. 2008. Walking the dog: Is pet ownership associated with physical activity in California? *Journal of Physical Activity and Health* 5(2):216-28.

Ye, Z., and H. Song. 2008. Antioxidant vitamin intake and risk of coronary heart disease: A meta-analysis of cohort studies. *European Journal of Cardiovascular Prevention and Rehabilitation* 15(1):26-34.

9. NUTRITION TO PREVENT AND TREAT CANCER

American Cancer Society. 2009. Cancer facts and figures. http://www.cancer.org/docroot/STT/STT_0.asp.

Argiles, J. M. 2005. Cancer-associated malnutrition. *European Journal of Oncology Nursing* 9(Supplement 2):539-50.

Aso, Y., H. Akaza, T. Kotake, et al. 1995. Preventative effect of a Lactobacillus casei preparation on the recurrence of superficial bladder cancer in a double-blind trial. The BLP study group. *European Urology* 27:104-9.

Benavente-Garcia, O., and J. Castillo. 2008. Update on uses of citrus flavonoids: New findings in anticancer, cardiovascular and anti-inflammatory activity. *Journal of Agricultural and Food Chemistry* 56:6185-205.

Block, G., B. Patterson, and A. Subar. 1992. Fruit, vegetables and cancer prevention: A review of the epidemiological evidence. *Nutrition and Cancer* 18:1-29.

LUKE CURTIS, MD

Carpenter, C. L., M. C. Yu, S. J. London. 2009. Dietary isothiocyanates, glutathione S-transferase M1 (GSTM1), and lung cancer risk in African Americans and Caucasians from Los Angeles County, California. *Nutrition and Cancer* 61(4):492-9.

Chan, J. M., C. N. Holick, M. F. Leitzmann, et al. 2006. Diet after diagnosis and the risk of prostate cancer progression, recurrence and deaths (United States). *Cancer Causes and Control* 17:199-208.

Clarke, J. D.,R. H. Dashwood, and E. Ho. 2008. Multi-targeted prevention of cancer by sulforaphane. *Cancer Letters* 269(2):291-304.

Dewys, W., C. Begg, P. Lavin, et al. 1980. Prognostic effect of weight loss prior to chemotherapy in cancer patients. *American Journal of Medicine* 69:491-7.

Divisi, D., S. Di Tommaso, S. Salvemini, et al. 2006. Diet and cancer. *Acta Biomedica* 77:118-23.

Donaldson, M. S. 2004. Nutrition and cancer: A review of the evidence for an anti-cancer diet. *Nutrition Journal* 3:19-30.

Doyle, C., L. H. Kushi, T. Byers, et al. 2006. Nutrition and physical activity during and after cancer treatment: An American Cancer Society guide for informed choices. *CA Cancer Journal for Clinicians* 56:323-53.

Duncan, A. 2004. The role of nutrition in the prevention of breast cancer. *AACN Clinical Issues: Advanced Practice in Acute and Critical Care* 15(1):119-35.

Gallicchio, L., K. Boyd, G. Matanoski, et al. 2008. Carotenoids and risk of developing lung cancer: A systematic review. *American Journal of Clinical Nutrition* 88:372-83.

Garland, C. F., W. B. Grant, S. B. Mohr, et al. 2007. What is the dose-response relationship between vitamin D and cancer risk? *Nutrition Reviews* (1):S91-S95.

Ginde, A. A., M. C. Liu, C. A. Carlos, et al. 2009. Demographic differences and trends of vitamin D insufficiency in the US population. *Archives of Internal Medicine* 169(9):626-32.

Gonzalez, A., U. Peters, J. W. Lampe, and E. White. 2009. Zinc intake from supplements and diet and prostate cancer. *Nutrition and Cancer* 6(2):206-15.

Hartman, T. J., P. S. Albert, K. Synder, et al. 2005. The association of calcium and vitamin D and the risk of colorectal adenomas. *Journal of Nutrition* 135:252-9.

Haseen, F., M. M. Cantwell, J. M. O'Sullivan, and L. J. Murray LJ. 2009. Is there a benefit from lycopene supplementation in men with prostate cancer? A systematic review. *Prostate Cancer and Prostatic Diseases* 12:325-32.

Heber, D. 2008. Multitargeted therapy of cancer by ellagitannins. *Cancer Letters* 269:262-8.

Lamm, D., D. Riggs, J. Shriver J, et al. 1994. Megadose vitamins in bladder cancer: A double blind clinical trial. *Journal of Urology* 151:21-6.

Lanza, E., T. J. Hartman, P. S. Albert, et al. 2006. High dry bean intake and reduced risk of advanced colorectal adenoma

LUKE CURTIS, MD

recurrence among participants in the polyp prevention trial. *Journal of Nutrition* 136:1896-903.

Martinez, M. E., E. Ciovannucci, R. Jiang, et al. 2006. Folate fortification, plasma folate, homocysteine and colorectal cancer recurrence. *International Journal of Cancer* 119:1440-6.

Mathew, A., R. Sinha, R. Burt, et al. 2004. Meat intake and recurrence of colorectal adenomas. *European Journal of Cancer Prevention* 13:159-64.

May, P. E., A. Barber, J. T. O'Olimpico, et al. 2002. Reversal of cancer-related wasting using oral supplementation with a combination of beta-hydroxy-beta-methylbutyrate, arginine and glutamine. *American Journal of Surgery* 183:471-9.

McCarthy, D. O. 2003. Rethinking nutritional support for persons with cancer cachexia. *Biological Research in Nursing* 5:3-17.

McCue, P., and K. Shetty. 2004. Health benefits of soy isoflavonoids and strategies for enhancement: a review. *Current Reviews in Food Science and Nutrition* 44:361-7.

Medicine Net. 2010. Lung cancer. http://www.medicinenet.com/lung_cancer/article.htm.

Meyerhardt, J. A., D. Niedzwiecki, D. Hollis, et al. 2007. Association of dietary patterns with cancer recurrence and survival in patients with stage III colon cancer. *Journal of the American Medical Association* 298:754-64.

Milner, J. A. 2002. Strategies for cancer prevention: The role of diet. *British Journal of Nutrition* 87(Supplement 2):S65-S72.

Nagle, C. M., D. M. Purdie, P. M. Webb, et al. 2003. Dietary influences on survival after ovarian cancer. *International Journal of Cancer* 106:264-9.

Pierce, J. P., L. Natarajan, B. J. Caan, et al. 2007. Influence of a diet very high in vegetables, fruit and fiber and low in fat on prognosis following treatment of breast cancer. *Journal of the American Medical Association* 298:289-98.

Rock, C. L., S. W. Flatt, L. Natarajan, et al. 2005. Plasma carotenoids and disease-free survival in women with a history of breast cancer. *Journal of Clinical Oncology* 23:6631-8.

Seeram, N. P. 2008. Berry fruits for cancer prevention: Current status and future prospects. *Journal of Agricultural and Food Chemistry* 56:630-5.

Shukla, Y., and N. Kalra. 2007. Cancer chemoprevention with garlic and its constituents. *Cancer Letters* 247:167-181.

Skuladottir, H., A. Tjoenneland, K. Overvad, et al. 2006. Does high intake of fruit and vegetables improve lung cancer survival? *Lung Cancer* 51:267-73.

Udenigwe, C. C., V. R. Ramprasath, R. E. Aluko, and J. Jones. 2008. Potential of resveratrol in cancer and anti-inflammatory therapy. *Nutrition Reviews* 66(8):445-54.

Zhou, W., R. S. Heist, G. Liu, et al. 2007. Circulating 25-hydroxyvitamin D levels predict survival in early-stage non-small-cell lung cancer patients. *Journal of Clinical Oncology* 25:479-85.

LUKE CURTIS, MD

10. NUTRITION TO IMPROVE EYESIGHT

Age-Related Eye Disease Study Research Group (AREDS). 2001. A randomized, placebo-controlled, clinical trial of high-dose supplementation with vitamins C and E, beta-carotene and zinc for age-related macular degeneration and vision loss: AREDS report no. 8. *Archives of Ophthalmology* 119:1417-36.

Canter, P. H., and E. Ernst. 2004. Anthocyanosides of Vaccinum myrtillus (bilberry) for night vision: A systematic review of placebo-controlled trials. Surveys in Ophthalmology 49(1):38-50.

Cheng, Y. J., E. W. Greg, L. S. Geiss, et al. 2009. Association of hemoglobin A1C and plasma glucose levels in diabetic retinopathy prevalence in the US population. *Diabetes Care* 32(11):2027-32.

Coleman, A. L., R. L. Seitzman, S. R. Cummings, et al. 2009. The association of smoking and alcohol use with age related macular degeneration in the oldest old. *American Journal of Ophthalmology* In Press.

Delcourt, C., I. Carriere, A. Ponton-Sanchez, et al. 2001. Light exposure and the risk of age related macular degeneration: The Pathologies Oculaiers Liees a l-Age (POLA) study. *Archives of Ophthalmology* 119(10):1463-8.

Eye Digest. 2009. University of Illinois at Chicago Eye and Ear Infirmary. http://www.agingeye.net/maculardegen/maculardegeninformation.php.

Feher, J., B. Kovacs, I. Kovacs, et al. 2005. Improvement of visual functions and fundus alterations in early age-related macular degeneration treatment with a combination of acetyl-L-carnitine, n-3 fatty acids, and coenzyme Q_{10}. *Ophthalmologica* 219:154-66.

Jacques, P. F., A. Taylor, S. Moeller, et al. 2005. Long-term nutrient intake and 5-year change in nuclear lens opacities. *Archives of Ophthalmology* 123:517-24.

Lindblad, B. E., N. Hakansson, H. Svensson, et al. 2005. Intensity of smoking and smoking cessation in relation to risk of cataract formation: A prospective study for men. *American Journal of Epidemiology* 162(1):73-9.

Moeller, S., A. Taylor, K. Tucker, et al. 2004. Overall adherence of the Dietary Guidelines for Americans is associated with reduced prevalence of early age-related nuclear lens opacities in women. *Journal of Nutrition* 134:1812-9.

Neale, R. E., J. L. Purdie, L. W. Hirst, and A. C. Green. 2003. Sun exposure as a risk factor for nuclear cataract. *Epidemiology* 14(6):707-12.

Pelletier, A., J. Thomas, and F. Shaw. 2009. Vision loss in older persons. *American Family Physician* 79(11):963-70.

Pokhrel, A. K., K. R. Smith, A. Khalakdina, et al. 2005. Case-control study of indoor cooking exposure and cataract in Nepal and India. *International Journal of Epidemiology* 34(3):702-3.

Raniga, A., and M. J. Elder. 2009. Dietary supplement use in the prevention of age-related macular degeneration progression. *New Zealand Medical Journal* 122:32-8.

SanGiovanni, J., E. Chew, E. Agron, et al. 2008. The relationship between dietary omega-3 long-chain fatty acid intake with incident

LUKE CURTIS, MD

age-related macular degeneration. *Archives of Ophthalmology* 126(9):1274-9.

Skylan, D. 1987. Vitamin A in human nutrition. *Progress in Foods and Nutritional Science* 11(1):39-55.

Tan, J., J. Wang, V. Flood, et al. 2008. Dietary antioxidants and long-term incidence of age related macular degeneration. *Ophthalmology* 115:334-41.

Wrong Diagnosis. 2009. Cataracts. http://www.wrongdiagnosis. com/c/cataracts/prevalence.htm.

11. NUTRITION TO PREVENT AND TREAT DEMENTIA, DEPRESSION, AND HEADACHES

Alpert, J. E., G. Papakostas, and D. Mischoulon. 2004. S-adenosyl-L-methionine (SAMe) as an adjunct for resistant major depressive disorder. *Journal of Clinical Psychopharmacology* 24: 661-4.

Balk, E., M. Chung, G. Raman, et al. 2006. B vitamins and berries and age related neurodegenerative disorders. *Evidence Reports of Technology Assessment* 134:1-161.

Biondi, D. 2003. Opoid resistance in chronic daily headaches. *Current Pain and Headache Reports* 7:67-75.

Blake, H. 2009. How effective are physical activity interventions for alleviating depressive symptoms in older people? A systematic review. *Clinical Rehabilitation* 23:873-887.

Bountziouka, V., E. Polychronopoulous, A. Zeimbekis, et al. 2009. Long-term fish intake is associated with less severe depressive symptoms among elderly men and women: The MEDISE (MEDiterannean Islands Elderly) epidemiology study. *Journal of Aging and Health* 21(6):864-80.

Brookmeyer, R., S. Gray, and C. Kawas. 1998. Projections of Alzheimer's disease in the United States and the public health impact of delayed disease onset. *American Journal of Public Health* 88:1337-42.

Clarkson-Smith, L., and A. A. Hartley. 1990. The game of bridge as an exercise in working memory and reasoning. *Journal of Gerontology* 45(6):P233-8.

Dosunmu, R., Wu, J., M. R. Basha, and N. H. 2007. Zawia NH. Environmental and dietary risk factors in Alzheimer's disease. *Expert Review of Neurotherapy* 7(7):887-900.

Engelhart, M. J., M. I. Geerlings, A. Ruitenberg, et al. 2002. Dietary intake of antioxidants and risk of Alzheimer's disease. *Journal of the American Medical Association* (*JAMA*) 287:3223-9.

Evans, R. W., and R. Couch. 2001. Orgasm and migraine. *Headache* 41(5):512-4.

Gallucci, M., P. Antuono, F. Ongaro, et al. 2009. Physical activity, socialization and reading in the elderly over the age of seventy: What is the relation to cognitive decline? *Archives of Gerontology and Geriatrics* 48:284-6.

Gariballa, S., and S. Forster. 2007. Effects of dietary supplements on depressive symptoms in older patients: A randomized double-blind placebo-controlled trial. *Clinical Nutrition* 26:545-51.

LUKE CURTIS, MD

Golub, N. I., P. C. Winters, and E. Van Wijngaarden. 2009. A population-based study of blood lead levels in relation to depression in the United States. *International Archives of Occupational and Environmental Health* In Press.

Grunebaum, M. F., M. A. Oquendo, and J. A. Manly. 2008. Depressive symptoms and antidepressant use in a random community sample of ethnically diverse, urban elder persons. *Journal of Affective Disorders* 105(1-3):273-7.

Hartmann, R. E., E. Shah, A. M. Fagan, et al. 2006. Pomegranate juice decreases amyloid load and improves behavior in a mouse model of Alzheimer's disease. *Neurobiological Diseases* 24(3):506-15.

Hughes, T. F., R. Andel, B. J. Small, et al. 2009. Midlife fruit and vegetable consumption and risk of dementia in later life in Swedish twins. *American Journal of Geriatric Psychiatry* In Press.

Irving, G. F., Y. Freund-Levi, M. Eriksdottir-Jonhagen, et al. 2009. Omega-3 fatty acid supplementation effects on weight and appetite in patients with Alzheimer's disease: The omega-3 Alzheimer's Disease Study. *Journal of the American Geriatric Society* 57:11-7.

Jones, R. N., E. R. Marcantonio, and T. Rabinowitz T. 2003. Prevalence and correlates of recognized depression in US nursing homes. *Journal of the American Geriatric Society* 51(10):1404-9.

Joseph, J. A., N. A. Denisova, G. Arendash, et al. 2003. Blueberry supplementation enhances signaling and prevents behavioral deficits in an Alzheimer's disease model. *Nutritional Neuroscience* 6(3):153-62.

Joseph, J. A., B. Shukitt-Hale, and L. M. Willis. 2009. Grape juice, berries and walnuts affect brain aging and behavior. *Journal of Nutrition* 139:1813-7S.

Koenig, H. C. 2009. Research on religion, spirituality, and mental health, a review. *Canadian Journal of Psychiatry* 54(5):283-91.

Krikorian, R., T. A. Nash, M. D. Shidler, et al. 2009. Concord grape juice supplementation improves memory function in older adults with mild cognitive impairment. *British Journal of Nutrition* In Press.

Krikorian, R., M. D. Shidler, T. A. Nash, et al. 2010. Blueberry supplementation improves memory in older adults. *Journal of Agricultural and Food Chemistry* In Press.

Larson, J. 1992. *Alcoholism: The biochemical connection. Chapter on good-bye depression.* Random House. http://www.trans4mind.com/nutrition/depression.html.

Lin, P. Y., and K. P. Su. 2007. A meta-analytic review of double-blind, placebo-controlled trials of the antidepressant efficacy of omega-3 fatty acids. *Journal of Clinical Psychiatry* 68(7):1056-61.

Lindenbaum, J., I. Rosenberg, P. Wilson, et al. 1994. Prevalence of cobalmin deficiency in the Framingham elderly population. *American Journal of Clinical Nutrition* 60:2-11.

Martin, R., and C. Becker. 1993. Headaches from chemical exposures. *Headache* 33:555-9.

Miller, A. L. 1998. St. John's wort (Hypericum perforatum): Clinical effects on depression and other conditions. *Alternative Medicine Review* 3(1):18-26.

LUKE CURTIS, MD

Millichap, G., and M. Vee. 2003. The diet factor in pediatric and adult migraine. *Pediatric Neurology* 28:9-15.

Morris, M. C., D. E. Evans, J. L. Bienias, et al. 2003. Consumption of fish and n-3 fatty acids and risk of incident Alzheimer's disease. *Archives of Neurology* 60:940-6.

Morris, M. C. 2009. The role of nutrition in Alzheimer's disease: Epidemiological evidence. *European Journal of Neurology* 16(Supplement 1):1-7.

Narin, S. O., and L. Pinar. 2003. The effects of exercise and exercise-related changes in blood nitric oxide level on migraine headache. *Clinical Rehabilitation* 17:624-30.

Norton, M. C., A. Singh, I. Skoog, et al. 2006. Church attendance and new episodes of major depression in a community of older adults. *Journal of Gerontology B Psychological Sciences and Social Sciences* 63(3):P129-37.

Oudshoorn, C., F. U. Mattace-Raso, N. Van Der Velde, et al. 2008. Higher serum vitamin D levels are associated with better cognitive test performance in patients with Alzheimer's disease. *Dementia and Geriatric Cognitive Disorders* 25:539-43.

Perez, C. A, and J. M. Cancela Carral. 2008. Benefits of physical exercise for older adults with Alzheimer's disease. *Geriatric Nursing* 29(6):384-91.

Peres, M., E. Zuckerman, W. B. Young, and S. D. Silberstein. 2002. Fatigue in chronic migraine patients. *Cephalagia* 22(9):720-4.

Reinisch, V. M., C. J. Schankin, J. Felbinger, et al. 2008. Headache in the elderly. *Schmerz* 22(Supplement 1):22-30 (article in German).

Reyes-Ortiz, C. A., I. M. Berges, M. A. Raji, et al. 2008. Church attendance mediates the association between depressive symptoms and cognitive functioning among older Mexican Americans. *Journal of Gerontology: A Biological and Medical Sciences* 63(5):480-6.

Samieri, C., M. A. Jutland, C. Feart, et al. 2008. Dietary patterns derived by hybrid clustering method in older people: Association with cognition, mood, and self-rated health. *Journal of the American Dietetic Association* 108:1461-71.

Sandor, P. 2005. Efficacy of Coenzyme Q_{10} in migraine prophylaxis: A randomized controlled trial. *Neurology* 64(4):713-5.

Sarris, J., N. Schoendorfer, and D. J. Kavanagh. 2009. Major depressive disorder and nutritional medicine: A review of monotherapies and adjuvant treatments. *Nutrition Reviews* 67(3):125-31.

Scarmeas, N., J. A. Luchsinger, N. Schupf, et al. 2009. Physical activity, diet and risk of Alzheimer's disease. *Journal of the American Medical Association* 302(6):627-37.

Shenassa, E. D., C. Daskalakis, A. Liebhaber, et al. 2007. Dampness and mold in the home and depression: An examination of mold-related illness and perceived control of one's home as possible depression pathways. *American Journal of Public Health* 97(10):1893-7.

Smoliner, C., K. Norman, K. H. Wagner, et al. 2009. Malnutrition and depression in the institutionalized elderly. *British Journal of Nutrition* 102(11):1663-7.

LUKE CURTIS, MD

Stallones, L., and C. Beseler. 2002. Pesticide poisoning and depressive symptoms among farm residents. *Annals of Epidemiology* 12:389-94.

Toth, C. 2003. Medications and substances as a cause of headache: A systematic review of the literature. *Clinical Neuropharmacology* 26(3):122-36.

Times Online (London). September 8, 2005. Sudoku keeps brain younger. http://www.timesonline.co.uk/tol/news/uk/article564063.ece.

Turner, E. H., J. M. Loftis, and A. D. Blackwell. 2006. Serotonin a la carte: Supplementation with the serotonin precursor 5-hydroxytryptophan. *Pharmacology and Therapeutics* 109:325-38.

12. NUTRITION TO PREVENT AND TREAT DIABETES

Casas-Agustench, P., P. Lopez-Uriate, M. Bullo, et al. 2009. Effects of one serving of mixed nuts on serum lipids, insulin resistance and inflammatory markers in patients with the metabolic syndrome. *Nutrition, Metabolism and Cardiovascular Disease* In Press.

Cereda, E, A. Gini, C. Pedrolli, and A. Vanotti. 2009. Disease-specific, versus standard, nutritional support of pressure ulcers in institutionalized older adults: A randomized controlled trial. *Journal of the American Geriatric Society* 57:1395-402.

Chau, D., and S. B. Elderlman. 2001. Clinical management of diabetes in the elderly. *Clinical Diabetes* 19(4):172-5.

Chu, J. Bloodless diabetes monitoring. February 27, 2008. http://technologyreview.com/biomedicine/20343/.

Goyal, S. K., S. Samsher, and R. K. Goyal. 2009. Stevia: A biosweetener: A review. *International Journal of Food Science and Nutrition* In Press.

Jiang, R., J. E. Manson, M. J. Stampfer, et al. Nut and peanut butter consumption and risk of type 2 diabetes in women. *Journal of the American Medical Association* 288(20):2554-60.

Khaw, K. T., and N. Wareham. 2006. Glycated hemoglobin as a marker of cardiovascular risk. *Current Opinion in Lipidology* 17(6):637-43.

Li, W. L., H. C. Zheng, J. Bukuru, and N. De Kimpe. 2004. Natural medicines used in traditional Chinese medical system for therapy of diabetes mellitus. *Journal of Ethnopharmacology* 92: 1-21.

Liu, S., M. Serdula, and S. J. Janket. 2004. A prospective study of fruit and vegetable intake and risk of type 2 diabetes in women. *Diabetes Care* 27(12):2993-6.

Ludvik, B., M. Hanefeld, and G. Pacini. 2008. Improved metabolic control by Ipomoea batatas is associated with increased adinectin and decreased fibrinogen levels in type 2 diabetic subjects. *Diabetes, Obesity and Metabolism* 10(7):586-92.

Magkos, F., M. Yannakoulia, J. L. Chen, and C. S. Mantzoros. 2009. Management of the metabolic syndrome and type 2 diabetes through lifestyle management. *Annual Reviews of Nutrition* 29:223-56.

LUKE CURTIS, MD

Martineau, L., A. Couture, and D. Spoor. 2006. Anti-diabetic properties of the Canadian lowbush blueberry Vaccinium augustifolium. *Phytomedicine* 13:612-23.

McCue, P., Y. I. Kwon, and K. Shetty. 2005. Anti-diabetic and anti-hypertensive potential of sprouted and solid state bioprocessed soybean. *Asia Pacific Journal of Clinical Nutrition* 14(2):145-52.

Meyer, K. A., L. Kushi, D. R. Jacobs, et al. 2000. Carbohydrates, dietary fiber, and incident type 2 diabetes in older women. *American Journal of Clinical Nutrition* 71:921-30.

Mole, P. 1990. Impact of energy intake and exercise on metabolic rate. *Sports Medicine* 10(2):72-87.

Nahas, R., and M. Moher. 2009. Complimentary and alternative medicine for the treatment of type 2 diabetes. *Canadian Family Physician* 55(6):591-6.

Ord, H. 2007. Nutritional support for patients with infected wounds. *British Journal of Nursing* 16:21:1346-52.

Rost, K. M., K. S. Flavin, L. E. Schmidt, and J. B. McGill. 1990. Self-care predictors of metabolic control in NIDDM patients. *Diabetes Care* 13(11):1111-3.

Sheela, C. G., K. Kumud, and K. T. Augusti. 1995. Anti-diabetic effects of onion and garlic sulfoxide amino acids in rats. *Planta Medicina* 61(4):356-7.

Stechschulte, B. A., R. S. Kirsner, and D. G. Federman. 2009. Vitamin D: Bone and beyond, rationale and recommendation for supplementation. *American Journal of Medicine* 122:793-802.

Sumpio, E. A., J. Aruny, and P. A. Blume. 2004. The multidisciplinary approach to limb salvage. *Acta Chir Belgium* 104(6):647-53.

Suppapitiporn, S., N. Kanpalso, and S. Suppapitiporn. 2006. The effect of cinnamon cassie powder in type 2 diabetes patients. *Journal of the Medical Association of Thailand* 89(Supplement 3):S200-5.

Web MD, Diabetes Health Center. 2009. http://diabetes.webmd. com/.

Whitney, E., and S. R. Rolfes. 2008. *Understanding nutrition.* 11th ed. Belmont, California: Thomas Wadsworth.

Vaquero, M. P. 2002. Magnesium and trace elements in the elderly: Intake, status and recommendations. *Journal of Nutrition, Health and Aging* 6(2):147-53.

13. NUTRITION TO PREVENT AND TREAT DIGESTIVE PROBLEMS

Bakos, N., I. Scholl, K. Szalai, et al. 2006. Risk assessment in elderly for sensitization to food and respiratory allergens. *Immunology Letters* 107:15-21.

Bennett, W. G., and J. J. Cerda. 1996. Benefits of dietary fiber. *Postgraduate Medicine* 99(2):153-6, 166-8.

Bijkerk, C. J., N. J. De Wit, J. V. M. Muris, et al. 2009. Soluble or insoluble fibre in irritable bowel syndrome in primary care? Randomised placebo controlled trial. *British Medical Journal* (*BMJ*) 339:b3154-61.

LUKE CURTIS, MD

Chmielewska, A., and H. Szajewska. 2010. Systemic review of randomized controlled trials: Probiotics for functional constipation. *World Journal of Gastroenterology* 16(1):69-75.

Cook, S. I., and J. H. Sellin. 1998. Review article: Short chain fatty acids in health and disease. *Alimentary Pharmacological Therapy* 12:499-507.

Crane, S. J., and N. J. Talley. 2007. Chronic gastrointestinal symptoms in the elderly. *Clinics in Geriatric Medicine* 23:721-34.

DeLegge, M. H. 2008. Enteral feeding. *Current Opinion in Gastroenterology* 24(2):184-9.

Drisko, J., B. Bischoff, M. Hall, and R. McCallum. 2006. Treating irritable bowel syndrome with a food elimination diet followed by food challenge and probiotics. *Journal of the American College of Nutrition* 25(6):514-22.

Groce, V. Jan. 31, 2008. About.com Food Allergies. Can I take Christian Holy Communion if I have a wheat allergy or celiac disease? http://foodallergies.about.com/od/wheatallergies/f/communionwheat.htm.

Heidelbaugh, J. J., T. T. Nostrant, C. Kim, and R. Van Harrison. 2003. Management of gastroesophageal reflux disease. *American Family Physician* 68(7):1311-8.

Hilton, E., H. D. Isenberg, P. Alperstein, et al. 1992. Ingestion of yogurt containing Lactobacillus acidophilus as prophylaxis for candidal vaginitis. *Annals of Internal Medicine* 116(5): 353-7.

Lee, S. Y., Y. W. Shin, and K. B. Hahm. 2008. Phytoceuticals: Mighty but ignored weapons against Helicobacter pylori infection. *Journal of Digestive Diseases* 8:129-39.

Mayo Clinic. 2009. Irritable bowel syndrome. http://www. mayoclinic.com/health/irritable-bowel-syndrome/DS00106/ DSECTION=lifestyle-and-home-remedies.

Nikfar, S., R. Rahimi, F. Rahimi, et al. 2008. Efficacy of probiotics in irritable bowel syndrome: A meta-analysis of randomized controlled trials. *Diseases of Colon and Rectum* 51:1775-80.

Ramakrishnan, K., and R. C. Salinas. 2007. Peptic ulcer disease. *American Family Physician* 76:1005-12.

Rashtak, S., and J. A. Murray. 2009. Celiac disease in the elderly. *Gastroenterology Clinics of North America* 38:433-46.

Salzman, H., and D. Lillie. 2005. Diverticular disease: Diagnosis and treatment. *American Family Physician* 72:1229-34.

Stacewicz-Sapuntzakis, M., P. E. Bowen, E. A. Hussain, et al. 2001. Chemical composition of potential health effects of prunes: A functional food? *Critical Reviews in Food Science and Nutrition* 41(4):251-86.

Yalcin, A. S. 2006. Emerging therapeutic potential of whey proteins and peptides. *Current Pharmaceutical Design* 12:1637-43.

LUKE CURTIS, MD

14. NUTRITION TO PREVENT AND TREAT KIDNEY FAILURE

Akgul, A., A. Bilgic, and S. Sezer. 2007. Effect of protein-energy malnutrition on erythropoietin requirements in maintenance hemodialysis patients. *Hemodialysis International* 11:198-203.

Arora, P. 2009. Verrelli. Chronic renal failure. eMedicine. http://emedicine.medscape.com/article/238798-overview.

Bamonti-Catena, F., G. Buccianti, and A. Porcella. 1999. Folate measurements in patients on regular hemodialysis treatment. *American Journal of Kidney Disease* 33:492-7.

Berne, R. M., and M. N. Levy. 2008. *Physiology*. 4th ed. St. Louis, Missouri: Mosby.

Cabral, P. C., A. S. Diniz, and I. K. De Arruda. 2005. Vitamin A and zinc status in patients on maintenance hemodialysis. *Nephrology* (Carlton) 10:459-63.

Chandna, S. M., J. E. Tattersall, and G. Nevett. 1997. Low serum vitamin B$_{12}$ levels in chronic high-flux hemodialysis patients. *Nephron* 76:259-63.

Cianciaruso, B., G. Brunori G, and J. D. Kopple. 1995. Cross-sectional comparison of malnutrition in continuous ambulatory peritoneal dialysis and hemodialysis patients. *American Journal of Kidney Disease* 26:475-86.

Clements, L., and I. Ashurst. 2006. Dietary Strategies to halt the progression of chronic kidney disease. *EDTNA Journal* 32(4):192-7.

Cusumano, A., M. Lombardo, C. Milano, et al. 1996. Nutritional status of patients on chronic hemodialysis. *Medicina* (Buenos Aires) 56:643-9 (article in Spanish).

Debska-Slizien, A., A. Kawecka, and K. Wojnarowski. 2007. Carnitine content in different muscles of patients receiving maintenance hemodialysis. *Journal of Renal Nutrition* 17: 275-81.

Fehrman-Ekholm, I., A. Lotsander, et al. 2008. Concentrations of vitamins C, vitamin B_{12} and folic acid in patients treated with hemodialysis and online hemodifiltration or hemofiltration. *Scandinavian Journal of Urology and Neprhology* 42(1):74-80.

Friedman, A., and S. Moe. 2006. Review of the effects of omega-3 supplementation in dialysis patients. *Clinical Journal of the American Society of Nephrology* 1:182-92.

Guarnieri, G., G. Biolo, P. Vinci, et al. 2007. Advances in carnitine in chronic uremia. *Journal of Renal Nutrition* 17:23-9.

Handelman, G. J. 2007. Vitamin C deficiency in dialysis patients: Are we perceiving the tip of an iceberg? *Nephrology, Dialysis and Transplantation* 22:328-31.

Heldal, K., A. Hartmann, D. C. Grootendorst, et al. 2009. Benefit of kidney transplantation beyond 70 years of age. *Nephrology, Dialysis and Transplantation* In Press.

Higuchi, T., Y. Matsukawa, and K. Okada. 2006. Correction of copper deficiency improves erythropoetin unresponsiveness in hemodialysis patients with anemia. *Internal Medicine* 45:271-3.

LUKE CURTIS, MD

Hung, S. C., S. H. Hung, D. C. Tarng, et al. 2001. Thiamine deficiency and unexplained encephalopathy in hemodialysis and peritoneal dialysis patients. *American Journal of Kidney Disease* 38:941-7.

Johnson, D. W., C. A. Pollock, and I.C. MacDougall. 2007. Erythropoiesis-stimulating agent hyporesponsiveness. *Nephrology* (Carlton) 12:321-30.

Keven, K., S. Kutley, G. Nergizoglu, and S. Erturk. 2003. Randomized, crossover study of the effect of vitamin C on EPO response in hemodialysis patients. *American Journal of Kidney Disease* 41:1233-9.

Kopple, J. D. 2001. The National Kidney Foundation K/DOQI clinical practice guidelines for dietary protein intake for chronic dialysis patients. *American Journal of Kidney Disease* 38(4 Supplement 1):S68-S72.

LaClair, R. E., R. N. Hellman, and S. L. Karp. 2005. Prevalence of calcidiol deficiency in CKD:A cross-sectional study across latitudes in the United States. *American Journal of Kidney Disease* 45:1026-33.

Melamed, M. L., B. Astor, E. D. Michos, et al. 2009. 23-hydroxyvitamin D levels, race, and the progression of kidney disease. *Journal of the American Society of Nephrology* 20(12):2631-9.

Naughton, C. 2008. Drug-induced nephrotoxicity. *American Family Physician* 78(6):743-50.

Perunicic-Pekovic, G. B., Z. R. Rasic, and S. I. Pljesa. 2007. Effect of n-3 fatty acids on nutritional status and inflammatory markers in haemodialysis patients. *Nephrology* (Carlton) 12:331-6.

Robertson, L., N. Waugh, and A. Robertson. 2007. Protein restriction for diabetic renal disease. *Cochrane Database Syst Rev* 17:CD002181.

Sen, D., and J. Prakash. 2000. Nutrition in dialysis patients. *Journal of the Associations of Physicians in India* 48:724-30.

Singh, J., H. K. Khanna, and M. A. Niaz. 2000. Randomized, double-blind placebo-controlled trial of coenzyme Q_{10} in chronic renal failure: Discovery of a new role. *Journal of Nutrition and Environmental Medicine* 10:281-8.

Snyder, S., and B. Pendergraph. 2005. Detection and evaluation of chronic kidney disease. *American Family Physician* 72:1723-34.

Svensson, M., E. B. Schmidt, K. A. Jorgensen, and J. H. Christensen. 2006. N-3 fatty acids as secondary prevention against cardiovascular events in patients who undergo chronic hemodialysis: A randomized, placebo-controlled intervention trial. *Clinical Journal of the American Society of Nephrology* 1:780-6.

Teng, M., W. Wolf, and M. N. Ofsthun. 2005. Activated injectable vitamin D and hemodialysis survival: A historical cohort study. *Journal of the American Society of Nephrology* 16:1115-25.

Triolo, L., S. Lippa, A. Oradei, P. De Sole, and R. Mori. 1994. Serum coenzyme Q_{10} in uremic patients on chronic hemodialysis. *Nephron* 66:153-6.

LUKE CURTIS, MD

15. NUTRITION AND CHONIC FATIGUE, FIBROMYALGIA, AND SLEEP PROBLEMS

Al-Lawati, N. M., S. R. Patel, and N. T. Ayas. 2009. Epidemiology, risk factors, and consequences of obstructive sleep apnea and short sleep duration. *Progress in Cardiovascular Disease* 51(4):285-93.

Almeida, F. R., and A. A. Lowe. 2009. Principles of oral appliance therapy for the management of snoring and sleep disordered breathing. *Oral and Maxillofacial Surgery Clinics of North America* 21(4):413-20.

Bannwarth, B., F. Blotman, K. Roue-Le Lay, et al. 2009. Fibromyalgia syndrome in the general population of France: A prevalence study. *Joint, Bone and Spine* 76:184-7.

Barbe, F., J. Sunyer, A. De La Pena, et al. 2007. Effect of continous positive airway pressure and the risk of road accidents in sleep apnea patients. *Respiration* 74(1):44-9.

Behan, P. O., W. H. Behan, and D. Horrobin. 1990. Effect of high dose essential fatty acids on the postviral fatigue syndrome. *Acta Neurologica Scandinavia* 82(3):209-16.

Birdsall, T. C. 1998. 5-Hydroxytryptophan: A clinically effective serotonin precursor. *Alternative Medicine Review* 3(4):271-80.

Bou-Holaigah, I., P.C. Rowe, J. Kan, and H. Calkins. 1995. The relationship between neutrally mediated hypotension and the chronic fatigue syndrome. *Journal of the American Medical Association (JAMA)* 274(12):961-7.

Bratton, R. L., and G. R. Corey. 2005. Tick-borne disease. *American Family Physician* 71:2323-32.

Buscemi, N., B. Vandermeer, and N. Hooton. 2005. The efficacy and safety of exogenous melatonin for primary sleep disorders. *Journal of General Internal Medicine* 20:1151-8.

Caldwell, K., G. A. Miller, R. Y. Wang, et al. 2008. Iodine status of the US population, National Health and Nutrition Examination Survey 2003-4. *Thyroid* 18(11):1207-14.

Crook, W. G. 1986. *The yeast connection.* 3rd ed. Jackson, Tennessee: Professional Books.

Dennis, D., D. Robertson, L. Curtis, and J. Black. 2009. Fungal exposure endocrinopathy in sinusitis with growth hormone deficiency: The Dennis Robertson syndrome. *Inhalation Toxicology* 25(9-10):669-680.

Flemons, W. W. 2002. Obstructive sleep apnea. *New England Journal of Medicine* 347(7): 498-504.

Guralnik, J., W. Ershler, S. Schrier, and V. Picozzi. 2005. Anemia in the elderly: A public health crisis in hematology. *American Society of Hematology* 528-532.

Hirshkowitz, M. 2008. The clinical consequences of obstructive sleep apnea and associated excessive sleepiness. *Journal of Family Medicine* 57(8):S9-S16.

Holistic Online. 2009. Alternative and integral therapies for insomnia. http://www.holistic-online.com/remedies/Sleep/sleep_ins_nutrition.htm.

LUKE CURTIS, MD

Hueston, W. J. 2001. Treatment of hypothyroidism. *American Family Physician* 64(10): 1717-24.

Jessop, C. May 26, 1989. Meeting Sheds light on chronic fatigue. *American Medical News.*

Karkoulias, K., P. Perimenis, N. Charokopos, et al. 2007. Does CPAP improve erectile dysfunction in patients with sleep apnea syndrome? *Clinical Therapeutics* 158(6):515-8.

Kaufmann, D. 2003. *The fungal link: Tracking the cause.* Volume 2. Rockwall, Texas: Mediatrition Publishers.

_____. 2008. *The fungus link.* Volume 1, 2nd series. Rockwall, Texas: Mediatrition Publishers.

_____. 2008. *The fungal link.* Volume 3, 2nd ed. Rockwall, Texas: Mediatrition Publishers.

King, A. C., R. F. Oman, G. S. Brassington, et al. 1997. Moderate-intensity exercise and self-reported quality of sleep in older adults. A randomized controlled trial. *Journal of the American Medical Association* 277(1):32-7.

Liebermann, J. A. 2009. Obstructive sleep apnea (OSA) and excessive sleepiness associated with OSA: Recognition in the primary care setting. *Postgraduate Medicine* 121(4):33-41.

Maes, M., I. Mihaylova, M. Kubera, et al. 2009. Coenzyme Q_{10} deficiency in myalgic encephalomyelitis /chronic fatigue syndrome (ME/CFS) is related to fatigue, autonomic and neurocognitive symptoms and is another factor explaining the early mortality in ME/CFS due to cardiac complications. *Neuroendocrine Letters* In Press.

Malaguarmera, M., M. P. Gargante, E. Cristaldi, et al. 2008. Acetyl-L-carnitine (ALC) treatment in elderly patients with fatigue. *Archives of Geriatrics and Gerontology* 46(2):181-90.

MayoClinic.com. 2009. Insomnia: Are there foods that help you sleep better? http://www.mayoclinic.com/health/foods-that-help-you-sleep/AN01582.

Neubauer, D. N. 1999. Sleep problems in the elderly. *American Family Physician* 59(9): 2551-60.

Norman, D., and J. S. Loredo. 2008. Obstructive sleep apnea and older adults. *Clinical and Geriatric Medicine* 24:151-65.

Pall, M. 2009. *Multiple chemical sensitivity: Toxicological questions and mechanisms. General and applied toxicology.* 3rd ed. New York, London: John Wiley and Sons.

Parish, J. M., and P. J. Lyng. 2003. Quality of life in bed partners of patients with obstructive sleep apnea of hyponea after treatment with continuous positive airway pressure. *Chest* 124:942-7.

Russell, I. J., J. E. Michalek, J. D. Flechas, and G. E. Abraham. 1995. Treatment of fibromyalgia syndrome with Super Malic: A randomized, double-blind, placebo-controlled crossover pilot study. *Journal of Rheumatology* 22(5):953-8.

Siccoli, M. M., J. C. T. Pepperell, M. Kohler, et al. 2008. Effects of continuous positive airway pressure on quality of life in patients with moderate to severe obstructive sleep apnea. *Sleep* 31(11):1551-8.

Teitelbaum, J. E., B. Bird, R. M. Greenfield, et al. 2001. Effective treatment of chronic fatigue syndrome: A randomized,

LUKE CURTIS, MD

double-blind, placebo-controlled, intent to treat study. *Journal of Chronic Fatigue Syndrome* 8(2):3-28.

Theou, O., G. R. Jones, T. J. Overend, et al. 2008. An exploration of the association between frailty and muscle fatigue. *Applied Physiology, Nutrition and Metabolism* 33(4):651-665.

Timlin, M. T., and M. A. Pereira. 2007. Breakfast frequency and quality in the etiology of adult obesity and chronic diseases. *Nutrition Reviews* (1):268-81.

Tralongo, P., D. Respini, and F. Ferrau. 2003. Fatigue and aging. *Critical Reviews in Oncology/Hematology* 48 Supplement:S57-S64.

Viaene, M., G. Vermeir, and L. Godderis. 2009. Sleep disturbances and occupational exposure to solvents. *Sleep Medicine Reviews* 13:235-43.

Werbach, M. R. 2000. Nutritional strategies for treating chronic fatigue syndrome. *Alternative Medicine Review* 5(2):93-108.

Wick, J. Y., and J. LaFluer. 2007. Fatigue: Implications for the elderly. *Consulting Pharmacist 22(7):566-78.*

Yamamura, S., H. Morishima, and T. Kumano-go. 2009. The effect of Lactobacillus helveticus fermented milk on sleep and health perceptions in elderly subjects. *European Journal of Clinical Nutrition* 63(1):100-5.

Zias, N., V. Bezwada, S. Gilman S, and A. Chnroneou. 2009. Obstructive sleep apnea and erectile dysfunction: Still a neglected risk factor? *Sleep and Breathing* 13(1):3-10.

16. NUTRITION TO TREAT JOINT PROBLEMS

Castillo, R. C., M. J. Bosse, E. J. MacKenzie, and B. M. Patterson. 2005. Impact of smoking on fracture healing and risk of complications in limb-threatening open tibia fractures. *Journal of Orthopedic Trauma* 19:151-7.

Darlington, L., and N. Ramsey. 1991. Diets for rheumatoid arthritis. *Lancet* 338:1209.

Davies-Tuck, M., A. E. Wluka, A. Forbes, et al. 2009. Smoking is associated with increased cartilage loss and persistence of bone marrow lesions over 2 years in community-based individuals. *Rheumatology* 48:1227-31.

Efthimiou, P., and M. Kukar. 2009. Complementary and alternative medicine use in rheumatoid arthritis: Proposed mechanism of action and efficacy of common use used modalities. *Rheumatology International* In Press.

Fransen, M., and S. McConnell. 2008. Exercise for osteoarthritis of the knee. *Cochrane Database System Review* 8(4):CD004376.

Gregory, P., M. Sperry, and A. F. Wilson. 2008. Dietary supplements for osteoarthritis. *American Family Physician* 77(2):177-84.

Hatakka, K., J. Martio, M. Korpela, M. Herranen, T. Poussa, T. Laasanen, M. Saxelin, H. Vapaatalo, E. Molianen, and R. Korpela. 2003. Effects of probotic therapy on the activity and activation of rheumatoid arthritis: A pilot study. *Scandinavian Journal of Rheumatology* 32(4):211-5.

Hinman, R. S., and K. L. Bennell. 2009. Advances in insoles and shoes for knee osteoarthritis. *Current Opinion in Rheumatology* 21(2):164-70.

Hinton, R., R. L. Moody, A. W. Davis, and S. F. Thomas. 2002. Osteoarthritis: Diagnosis and therapeutic considerations. *American Family Physician* 65(5):841-8.

Khuder, S., A. Peshiman, and S. Agraharam. 2002. Environmental risk factors for rheumatoid arthritis. *Reviews in Environmental Health* 17(4):307-315.

Klippel, J. H., eds. 1997. *Primer on the rheumatic diseases.* Atlanta, Georgia: Arthritis Foundation.

Lieberman, A. 2003. Explosion of mold cases in homes, workplaces and occupational medicine practices. Presented at the 21st annual symposium on man and his environment, June 19-22, in Dallas, Texas.

Luosujarvi, T., T. Husman, and M. Seuri. 2003. Joint symptoms and diseases associated with moisture damage in a health center. *Clinical Rheumatology* 22(6):381-5.

Najm, W. I., S. Reinsch, F. Hoehler, et al. 2004. S-adenosylmethionine (SAMe) versus celoxicib for the treatment of osteoarthritis symptoms: A double-blind cross-over trial. *BMC Musculoskeletal Disorders* 5:6.

Rahmann, A. E., S. G. Brauer, and J. C. Nitz. 2009. A specific inpatient aquatic physiotherapy program improves strength after total hip or knee replacement surgery: A randomized controlled trial. *Archives of Physical Medicine and Rehabilitation* 90(5):745-55.

Richy, F., O. Bruyere, O. Ethgen, et al. 2003. Structural and symptomatic efficacy of glucosamine and chondroitin in knee osteoarthritis: A comprehensive meta-analysis. *Archives of Internal Medicine* 163(13):1514-22.

Smith, M. T., P. J. Quartana, R. M. Okonkwo, and A. Nasir. 2009. Mechanisms by which sleep disturbance contributes to osteoarthritis pain: A conceptual model. *Current Pain and Headache Reports* 13(6):447-54.

Stolt, P., H. Kallberg, and I. Lundberg. 2005. Silica exposure is associated with increased risk of developing rheumatoid arthritis: Results from the Swedish EIRA-study. *Annals of Rheumatic Disease* 64(4):582-6.

Taylor, D. H., V. Hasselblad, J. Henley, M. J. Thun, and F. A. Sloan. 2002. Benefits of smoking cessation for longevity. *American Journal of Public Health* 92:990-6.

17. NEAR-IDEAL DIETS: MENU GUIDELINES AND OTHER IDEAS TO IMPROVE ELDER NUTRIENT INTAKES.

Bradbury, J., J. M. Thomason, N. J. A. Jepson, et al. 2006. Nutrition counseling increases fruit and vegetable intake in the edentulous. *Journal of Dental Research* 85(5):463-8.

Brill, S., and E. Dean. 1994. *Identifying and harvesting edible and medicinal plants in wild (and not so wild) places.* New York City: Hearst Books.

Dannenberger, D., G. Nuernberg, N. Scollan, K. Ender, and K. Nuernberg. 2007. Diet alters the fatty acid composition of individual phospholipid classes in beef muscle. *Journal of Agricultural and Food Chemistry* 55(2):452-60.

De Oliveira, T. R. C., and M. L. M. A. Frigerio. 2004. Association between nutrition and the prosthetic condition in edentulous elderly. *Gerodontology* 21:205-8.

Douglass, C. W., A. Shih, and L. Ostry. 2002. Will there be a need for complete dentures in the United States in 2020? *Journal of Prosthetic Dentistry* 82:5-8.

Fraser, G. E., and D. J. Shavlik. 1997. Risk factors for all cause and coronary heart disease in the oldest old. The Adventist Health Study. *Archives of Internal Medicine* 157(19):2249-58.

Humbert, I. A., and J. A. Robbins. 2008. Dysphagia in the elderly. *Physical Medicine and Rehabilitation Clinics of North America* 19:853-66.

Hutton, B., J. Feine, and J. Morais. 2002. Is there an association between edentulism and nutritional state? *Journal of the Canadian Dietetic Association* 68(3):182-7.

Logemann, J. A. 2007. Swallowing disorders. *Best Practice Research in Clinical Gastroenterology* 21(4):563-73.

Mathey, M. F., V. Vanneste, C. De Graaf, L. De Groot, and W. Van Stavern. 2001. Health effect of improved meal ambience in a Dutch nursing home: 1 year intervention study. *Preventive Medicine* 32:416-23.

Mattes, R. D., P. M. Kris-Etherton, and G. D. Foster. 2008. Impact of peanuts and tree nuts on body weight and health weight loss in adults. *Journal of Nutrition* 138:1741S-1745S.

Quandt, S. A., H. Chen, R. A. Bell, et al. 2009. Food avoidance and food modification practices of older rural adults: association with oral health status and implications for service provision. *The Gerontologist* 50(1):100-11.

Qureshi, A. L., F. K. Suri, S. Ahmed, et al. 2007. Regular egg consumption does not increase the risk of stroke and cardiovascular disease. *Medical Science Monitor* 13(1):CR1-8.

Restani, P., A. Gaiaschi, A. Plebani, et al. 1999. Cross-reactivity between milk proteins from different animal species. *Clinical and Experimental Allergy* 29:997-1004.

Smith, A. 2002. Effects of caffeine on human behavior. *Food and Chemical Toxicology* 40: 1243-55.

Song, W. O., and J. M. Kerver. 2009. Nutritional contribution of eggs to American diets. *Journal of the American College of Nutrition* 19(5 Supplement):556S-562S.

Timlin, M. T., and M. A. Pereira. 2007. Breakfast frequency and quality in the etiology of adult obesity and chronic diseases. *Nutrition Reviews* (1):268-81.

Walls, A. W. G., and J. G. Steele. 2004. The relationship between oral health and nutrition in older people. *Mechanisms of Ageing and Development* 125:853-7.

Wild, C. P., and Y. Y. Gong. 2010. Mycotoxins and human disease: A largely ignored global health issue. *Carcinogenesis* 31(7):71-82.

Wright, L., M. Hickson, and G. Frost. 2006. Eating together is important: Using a dining room in an acute elderly medical ward increases energy intake. *Human Nutrition and Dietetics* 19:23-6.

LUKE CURTIS, MD

18. SUPPLEMENT SUGGESTIONS FOR SENIORS: WHY YOU NEED SUPPLEMENTS NOW EVEN IF YOU DID NOT NEED THEM IN MIDDLE AGE

All Experts. Scurvy: Encyclopedia. 2010. http://en.allexperts. com/e/s/sc/scurvy.htm.

Alonso, A., C. DeLaFunete, A. M. Martin-Arnau, et al. 2004. Fruit and vegetable consumption is inversely associated with blood pressure in a Mediterranean population with a high-vegetable-fat intake: The Seguimiento Universidad de Navarra (SUN) study. *British Journal of Nutrition* 92:311-9.

Baroja, M. L., P. V. Kirjavainen, S. Hekmat, and G. Reid. 2007. Anti-inflammatory effects of probiotic yogurt in inflammatory bowel patients. *Clinical and Experimental Immunology* 149: 470-9.

Bischoff-Ferrari, H. A., W. C. Willet, J. B. Wong, et al. 2009. Prevention of non-vertebral fractures with oral vitamin D and dose dependency. *Archives of Internal Medicine* 169(6):551-61.

Caso, G., P. Kelly, M. A. McNurlan, and W. E. Lawson. 2007. Effect of coenzyme Q_{10} on myopathic symptoms in patients treated with statins. *American Journal of Cardiology* 99(10): 1409-12.

Clark, R., G. Feleke, M. Din, et al. 2000. Nutritional treatment for acquired immunodeficiency virus-associated wasting using HMB, glutamine and arginine: A double-blind, placebo controlled study. *JPEN (Journal of Parenteral and Enteral Nutrition)* 24:133-9.

Clements, L., and I. Ashurst. 2006. Dietary strategies for halt the progression of chronic kidney disease. *EDTNA Journal* 32(4):192-7.

Curtis, L. 2008. Nutrition, copper and myelodysplasia. *Transfusion Medicine* 18:315-6.

Dannenberger, D., G. Nuernberg, N. Scollan, K. Ender, and K. Nuernberg. 2007. Diet alters the fatty acid composition of individual phospholipid classes in beef muscle. *Journal of Agricultural and Food Chemistry* 55(2):452-60.

DeLegge, M. H. 2008. Enteral feeding. *Current Opinion in Gastroenterology* 24(2):184-9.

eMEDTV, Niacin Flush. 2008. http://cholesterol.emedtv.com/niacin/niacin-flush.html.

Enache-Angoulvant, A., and C. Hennequin. 2005. Invasive Saccharomyces infection: A comprehensive review. *Clinical Infectious Diseases* 41(11):1559-68.

Etminan, M., J. M. Fitzgerald, M. Gleave, and K. Chambers. 2005. Intake of selenium in the prevention of prostate cancer: A systemic review and meta-analysis. *Cancer Causes and Control* 16:1125-31.

Fehrman-Ekholm, I., A. Lotsander, et al. 2008. Concentrations of vitamins C, vitamin B_{12} and folic acid in patients treated with hemodialysis and on-line hemodifiltration or hemofiltration. *Scandinavian Journal of Urology and Nephrology* 42(1):74-80.

Flores-Mateo, G., A. Navas-Acien, A. Pastor-Barriuso, and E. Guallar. 2006. Selenium and coronary heart disease: A meta-analysis. *American Journal of Clinical Nutrition* 84(4):762-73.

Fraser, J. July 5, 2005. Statistics prove prescription drugs are 16,400% more deadly than terrorists. *Natural News*. http://www.naturalnews.com/009278.html.

LUKE CURTIS, MD

Jacobs, E. T., R. Jiang, D. S. Alberts, et al. 2004. Selenium and colorectal adenoma: Results of a pooled analysis. *Journal of the National Cancer Institute* 96(22):1669-75.

Ginde, A. A., M. C. Liu, C. A. Carlos, et al. 2009. Demographic differences and trends of vitamin D insufficiency in the US population. *Archives of Internal Medicine* 169(9):626-32.

Gorelik, O., D. Almoznion-Sarafian, I. Feder, et al. 2003. Dietary intake of various nutrients in older patients with congestive heart failure. *Cardiology* 99:177-81.

Guralnik, J., W. Ershler, S. Schrier, and V. Picozzi. 2005. Anemia in the elderly: A public health crisis in hematology. *American Society of Hematology* 528-532.

Handelman, G. J. 2007. Vitamin C deficiency in dialysis patients: Are we perceiving the tip of an iceberg? *Nephrology, Dialysis and Transplantation* 22:328-31.

Hathcock, J. N., A. Shao, R. Vieth, and R. Heaney. 2007. Risk assessment for vitamin D. *American Journal of Clinical Nutrition* 85:6-18.

Hayes, A., and P. J. Cribb. 2008. Effect of whey protein isolate on strength, body composition and muscle hypertrophy during resistance training. *Current Opinion in Clinical Nutrition and Metabolic Care* 11(1):40-4.

Karppanen, H., and E. Mervaala. 2006. Sodium intake and hypertension. *Progress in Cardiovascular Disease* 9:59-75.

Kim, J. S., J. M. Wilson, and S. R. Lee. 2010. Dietary implications on mechanisms of sarcopenia: Roles of protein, amino acids and antioxidants. *Journal of Nutritional Biochemistry* In Press.

Keven, K., S. Kutley, G. Nergizoglu, and S. Erturk. 2003. Randomized, crossover study of the effect of vitamin C on EPO response in hemodialysis patients. *American Journal of Kidney Disease* 41:1233-9.

Kummerow, F. A. 2009. The negative effects of hydrogenated fats and what do about them. *Atherosclerosis* 205:458-65.

Lindenbaum, J., I. Rosenberg, P. Wilson, et al. 1994. Prevalence of cobalmin deficiency in the Framingham elderly population. *American Journal of Clinical Nutrition* 60:2-11.

Meunier, P. J., C. Roux, E. Seeman, et al. 2004. The effects of strontium ranelate on the risk of vertebral fracture in women with postmenopausal osteoporosis. *New England Journal of Medicine* 350:5:459-68.

Merck Online, 2007. Vitamin A. http://www.merck.com/mmpe/sec01/ch004/ch004g.html.

Miller, E. R., R. Pastor-Barriusco, D. Dalal, et al. 2005. Meta-analyses: High dosage vitamin E may increase all cause mortality. *Annals of Internal Medicine* 142(1):37-46.

Morris, M. C. 2009. The role of nutrition in Alzheimer's disease: Epidemiological evidence. *European Journal of Neurology* 16(Supplement 1):1-7.

Murray, M. 1996. *Encyclopedia of nutritional Supplements.* New York City: Three Rivers Press.

Nahas, R., and M. Moher. 2009. Complementary and alternative medicine for the treatment of type 2 diabetes. *Canadian Family Physician* 55(6):591-6.

LUKE CURTIS, MD

Natural Cures and Remedies. 2010. Natural cures for constipation. http://www.natural-cure-remedy.com/constipation.html.

Park, S., M. A. Johnson, and J. G. Fischer. 2008. Vitamin and mineral supplements: Barriers and challenges for older adults. *Journal of Nutrition for the Elderly* 27(3/4):297-317.

Prasad, A. S., J. T. Fitzgerald, J. W. Hess, et al. 1993. Zinc deficiency in elderly patients. *Nutrition* 9(3):218-24.

Radimer, K., B. Bindewald, J. Hughes, et al. 2004. Dietary supplement use by US adults: Data from the National Health and Nutrition Examination Survey, 1999-2000. *American Journal of Epidemiology* 160:339-49.

Raniga, A., and M. J. Elder. 2009. Dietary supplement use in the prevention of age-related macular degeneration progression. *New Zealand Medical Journal* 122:32-8.

Richy, F., O. Bruyere, O. Ethgen, et al. 2003. Structural and symptomatic efficacy of glucosamine and chondroitin in knee osteoarthritis: A comprehensive meta-analysis. *Archives of Internal Medicine* 163(13):1514-22.

Robotham, J. L., and P. S. Lietman. 1980. Acute iron poisoning. *American Journal of Diseases of Childhood* 134:875-9.

Rude, R. K., F. R. Singer, and H. E. Gruber. 2009. Skeletal and hormonal effects of magnesium deficiency. *Journal of the American College of Nutrition* 28(2):131-41.

Saul, A. FDA claims "food supplement" deaths; hides details from the Public. *Orthomolecular New Service.* http://www.orthomolecular.org/resources/omns/v04n13.shtml.

Samman, S., F. P. Kung, L. M. Carter, et al. 2009. Fatty acid composition of certified organic, conventional and omega-3 eggs. *Food Chemistry* 116:911-4.

Spence, J. D. 2006. Nutrition and stroke prevention. *Stroke* 37:2430-5.

Stechschulte, B. A., R. S. Kirsner, and D. G. Federman. 2009. Vitamin D: Bone and beyond, rationale and recommendation for supplementation. *American Journal of Medicine* 122:793-802.

Tang, B. M., G. D. Eslick, C. Nowson, et al. 2007. Use of calcium or calcium in combination with vitamin D supplementation to prevent fractures and bone loss in people aged 50 years and older: A meta-analysis. *Lancet* 370(9588):657-66.

Tiihonen, K., A. C. Ouwehand, and N. Rautonen. 2009. Human intestinal microbiota and healthy ageing. *Ageing Research Reviews* In Press.

Vaquero, M. P. 2002. Magnesium and trace elements in the elderly: Intake, status and recommendations. *Journal of Nutrition, Health and Aging* 6(2):147-53.

Whitney, E., and S. R. Rolfes. 2008. *Understanding nutrition.* Belmont, California: Thomson Wadsworth.

Wikipedia. 2010. Omega-3 fatty acid. http://en.wikipedia.org/wiki/Omega-3_fatty_acid.

Wintergerst, E. S., R. Maggini, and D. H. Hornig. 2007. Contribution of selected vitamins and trace elements to immune function. *Annals of Nutrition and Metabolism* 51:301-23.

LUKE CURTIS, MD

INDEX

B

bacteria
  bad. *See Closteridium difficile*
  friendly. *See* probiotic bacteria
  Lactobacillus, 71–72
  Lactobacillus casei, 122, 158,
    296
  Lactobacillus helviticus, 177
  Lactobacillus rhamnosus, 188
bad cholesterol. *See* cholesterol:
  low-density lipoprotein
bananas, 61, 82, 110, 166,
    196–97, 228, 239, 252, 255,
    257
Barrett's esophagus, 118
berries, 118
beta-carotene, 225
  consumption of, 116
beta-cryptoxanthin, 116
beta-hydroxy-beta-
    methylbutyrate, 49, 51, 122,
    299
Bifidobacterium, 72, 87–88, 107,
    158, 160, 204, 246–48
Bifidobacterium lactis, 158
bilberries, 129, 301
biotin, 229–30
bisphosphonates, 59
blood sugar control methods, 146
blueberries, 118, 134–35, 149,
    195–98, 252, 255, 278
blueberry juice, consumption of,
    135

BMI. *See* body mass index
body fat percentage,
    determination of, 39
body mass index range, 38
bone loss. *See* osteoporosis, 5,
    20, 40, 48, 57, 61–62, 64,
    66, 185, 229, 244, 274, 276,
    334
bone marrow, 75, 172
Borlaug, Norman, 17
boron, 244
Borrelia burgdorferi, 182
brain attack. *See* stroke
Brazil nuts, 72, 205, 244, 255,
    280
breakfast, 206
brewer's yeast, 225
British sailors, 231
broccoli, 60, 63, 72, 116-117, 123,
    127-128, 149, 156, 195-196,
    198-199, 203, 225-226, 228-229,
    231, 235, 237, 241, 252-255
buckwheat, 107, 160, 246
burn patients, 83
Bush, George, 39
butyric acid, gamma hydroxyl,
    214
Byrd, Robert, Jr., 16

C

cabbage, 63, 72, 116–17, 123,
    195–96, 199, 231, 235,
    253–54

LUKE CURTIS, MD

calcium, 59, 237–38

calorie, 24, 31, 45, 150, 172, 204, 251, 265

calories, 23–24, 28–31, 33, 39, 43, 48, 50, 61, 73, 75–76, 79, 82–83, 136–37, 172, 204–5, 207–8

cancer, 116, 120
  esophageal, 118, 155
  prevention of, 117–18

cancer patients, 41, 121

cancer-related malnutrition, 120–21

Candida, 182, 248

Candida diet, 182

Candida infection, 73, 159, 171, 182

cantaloupe, 63, 196, 199, 252

capillaries, 93

carbonated beverages, consumption of, 64

cardiovascular rehabilitation program, 99

carnitine, 100, 175, 220

carotenoids, 49, 61, 63, 123, 273, 298

carotid arteries, 103, 296

carrots, 199

cashews, 205, 255

cataracts, 126–29

Catheters, 90

cat's claw, 188

cauliflower, 117, 199, 254

celiac disease, 159–60, 313–14

centenarians, 14, 260

cheese, 42, 45, 49–50, 60, 72, 81, 141, 147, 175, 193, 196, 202–3, 205–6, 218, 225, 251–52

Chloride, 240

cholesterol
  high-density lipoprotein, 105, 242
  low-density lipoprotein, 105–8, 149, 204–5

Choline, 230

chondroitin sulfate, 186–87, 215, 236–37

chromium, 25, 147–48, 151, 243

chronic diarrhea, 28

chronic fatigue, 172–74, 176, 178, 181–83

chronic intestinal infections, 28

chronic obstructive pulmonary diseases, 113, 295

Churchill, Winston, 16

Cialis, 100

cinnamon, 149, 312

circadian rhythm, 177

cis confirmation, 222

citrus fruits, 61, 95, 110, 118, 166, 195, 231, 239, 267

Closeridium difficile, 28, 72, 87–88, 248

cobalmin, 228–29

cod-liver oil, 51, 60, 88, 98, 130, 202, 223, 225, 233, 253

coenzyme Q10, 30, 106, 175,

LUKE CURTIS, MD

docosahexaenoic acid, 222–23
donuts, commercial, 207
drugs, nutrient-depleting, 30, 109
dual energy x-ray absorptiometry
    scan, 58
Dual Energy X-Ray Absorption
    Scan, 58, 67
Dual Energy X-ray Scan, 58, 67
dwarf fruit trees, 199
dysphasia, 27

E

eating assistance, 102, 209
Echinacea, 74
edema, 41–42
eggs, 203
Eicosapentaenoic acid, 121,
    222–23
elderberry, 74
empty calories, 30
*Encyclopedia of Nutritional
    Supplements, The* (Murray),
    216
endorphins, 139
enteral feeding. *See* tube feeding
EPA. *See* eicosapentaenoic acid
ephedra, 214
erectile dysfunction, 100, 146,
    219–20, 289, 294, 321, 323
erythropoietin, 168
Escherichia coli, 158
esophageal cancer, 155
estrogen receptor modulators, 59

estrogen supplements, 59
exercise, 3, 5, 14, 17–18, 21,
    43–44, 47–48, 52–54,
    66–67, 98–99, 108, 139–40,
    149, 177–79, 183, 273–74
    mental, 139
    outdoor, 52
eyesight, failing, 125

F

fall prevention, 58
famous seniors, 16
fatigue, 75, 171, 173, 176, 181,
    225, 244, 286, 307, 321–23
Faust (von Goethe), 17
fiber, 31, 82, 106, 116, 148, 157,
    194–95, 204, 208
fibromyalgia, 171–72
Fieldler, Arthur, 17
filberts, 205, 255
fires, 83
fish, 29, 31, 33, 44, 48, 50–51, 53,
    60–62, 81, 100, 108, 121–23,
    127, 174–75, 201, 256
Fisher, Herbert, 19
Fisher, Zelmyra, 19
fish oil, 88–89, 112, 202
5-hydroxy tryptophan, 137
flax oil, 49, 108, 201
flu. *See* influenza
fludrocortisone, 174
fluoride, 62, 245–46
folate, 229

folic acid. *See* folate

food allergies, 159

food deserts, 29

free weights, 52

fruits, 33, 43–45, 50, 53, 61–62, 72, 95, 110, 113, 121–22, 126, 147, 188, 195, 197–98, 251–52

Fungus Link, The (Kaufmann), 183

G

gaining weight in underweight, 45

garlic, 73, 107

ginger, 111, 188

ginseng, 74, 100

glaucoma, 126, 150

glucosamine sulfate, 186, 236

glucose tolerance factor, 148, 243

gluten allergen. *See* celiac disease

goat's milk, 203

good cholesterol. *See* cholesterol: high-density lipoprotein

gorilla food, 196

grapes, 200

H

H1N1 swine flu, 69

Hamilton, Alice, 16

handwashing, 74–75, 90

hardening of arteries. *See* atherosclerosis

HDL. *See* cholesterol, high-density lipoprotein

headaches, 133, 140–42

heart, 93

heart attack (myocardial infarction), 96

heart attacks (myocardial infarction), 20, 95

heartburn, 28, 155–56

heart disease, 95, 99

heart failure, 95–97

Helicobacter, 73

hemodialysis, 165, 295, 316–17, 330

hemoglobin, 146, 240

hemoglobin A1C levels, 126, 146

hemp seed, 205

herbal seasonings, low-sodium, 110

hip fractures, 57

HMB. *See* beta-hydroxy-beta-methylbutyrate

homocysteine, 164, 294, 299

honeydew, 196, 199, 252

hospital-acquired infections, 69–70, 79–80, 89

hospital nutrition, 79

hypertension, 108–9, 163

hypotension, 110, 173

hypothyroidism, 176

I

IBS. *See* irritable bowel syndrome

immunonutrition enteral (tube

feeding) formulas, 86. *See also* tube feeding

impotence. *See* erectile dysfunction

infection and nutrition, 69–76

infection rates much higher among malnourished, 70

infections, 5–6, 20–21, 33–34, 69–70, 74–76, 79–82, 85–90, 112–13, 265–68, 270–71, 274–75, 277–81, 296–99, 306–10, 312–15, 332–34

influenza, 69

Inositol, 231

insomnia, 177, 185

insulin, 83, 145, 147

intermittent claudication, 104–5

intrinsic factor, 32

iodine, 174, 245

Irish moss, 200

iron, 240–41

irritable bowel syndrome, 28, 155, 157–59, 183, 312–14

isoflavone, 63, 119

isothiocyanates, consumption of, 117

J

Jenny Craig, 44

Jessop, Carol, 183

joint problems, 185

Jones, Mary Harris, 16

juice, 24, 117–18, 135, 157, 194, 206–7, 215, 251

Juice, 71

K

kale, 117, 127, 199, 226

Kaufmann, Doug, 183

Fungus Link, The, 183

kelp, 174, 193, 200, 241, 245, 252, 256

Kerry, John, 39

ketoconazole, 183

kidneys, 163

kidney transplantation, 165, 316

kiwi, 63, 195, 231

L

Lactobacillus, 204

laparoscopic surgery, 90

L-arginine, 220

L-carnitine, 76, 97–98, 100, 104, 128, 130, 166–68, 175–76, 215, 217, 219–20, 286, 316

LDL. *See* cholesterol: low-density lipoprotein

lecithin, 203

lettuce, 128, 195, 198, 200, 225, 235, 256

Lettuce, 253

Levitra, 100

L-glutamine, 220

limeys. *See* British sailors

linolenic acid, conjugated, 49

L-leucine, 221. *See also* beta-
    hydroxy-beta-methylbutyrate

low-sugar drinks, 82, 206

L-taurine, 220

lung cancer, 117, 205

lungs, 93

lutein, 127–29, 203

Lxodes scapularis. See deer tick

Lycopenes, 63, 117

Lyme disease, 182

M

Mack, Connie, 17

macula, 125

macular degeneration, 125,
    127–28, 130, 150, 219, 242,
    301, 303

magnesium, 61, 111, 113, 141,
    238

malic acid, 173

malnutrition, 70, 80–81, 102, 120

    extent of, 23

    obvious forms of, 23

    reasons for, 27

    not recognized or documented
        by physicians, 33

    and significantly higher infection
        rates associated with, 70

    very common in hospitalized
        seniors, 33

mammography, 115

Mandela, Nelson, 16

manganese, 244

Massine, Leonide, 89

Meals on Wheels, 209

meat, 43–44, 48, 61–62, 81, 141,
    147, 177, 182, 201–2

Meat, 252

meats, 53, 64

Meir, Golda, 16

melatonin, 177

methicillin-resistant *Staphylococcus
    aureus*, 69, 73

methionine, 72, 203, 216–17

milk, 111, 203–4

mitochondria, 175, 219, 235

mold exposure, 181–82, 287

Molybdenum, 246

monosodium glutamate, 141

monounsaturated fats, 221

Moses, Anna, 17

Mother Teresa, 17

MRSA. *See* methicillin-resistant
    Staphylococcus aureus

MSG. *See* monosodium
    glutamate

multiple organ failure syndrome, 85

Murray, Michael, 216

    *Encyclopedia of Nutritional
        Supplements, The*, 216

muscle loss. *See* sarcopenia

mycotoxins, 138, 164, 205, 328

myelodysplasia, 75–76, 277, 330

MyoVive, 97

N

LUKE CURTIS, MD

T

tea, 24, 81–82, 111, 121, 156, 194, 207, 235, 245, 251, 253–55

TENS, 188

thiamine, 226

thyroid problems, 133, 171, 176

tooth problems, 27

transcutaneous electrical nerve stimulation. See TENS

trauma patients, 83–85

triglycerides, 105–7

trimethoprim, 71, 279

tryptophan, 137

tube (enteral) feeding, 80, 84–85, 282, 313, 330

  death rates much lower among elders given prompt tube feeding, 84

  immunonutrition formulas greatly reduce infection rates, 86

type 1 diabetes. See diabetes: juvenile

type 2 diabetes. See diabetes: adult-onset

U

ulcers, 155–56

Uncommon Ground, 200

underweight, 5, 37–41, 45

  higher death rates in, 40

urinary tract infection, 71–72, 86, 278–79

US Department of Health and Human Services, 26, 267

UTI. See urinary tract infection

V

vacation travel, 18

vanadium, 246

vegetable consumption, 26, 62, 116–17

vegetables

  Allium family, 119, 195

  cruciferous, 117, 199

  vitamin K-containing, 62

veins, 103

Viagra, 19, 100

vitamin

  A, 224

  B complex, 173, 225

    B1. See thiamine, 230

    B2. See riboflavin, 230

    B3. See niacin, 230

    B5. See pantothenic acid

    B6. See pyridoxine, 230

    B12. See cobalmin, 230

  C, 25, 63, 96, 168, 231–32

  D, 49, 59–60, 232–33

    deficiency of, 233

  E, 96, 234

  K, 62, 235

von Goethe, Johann Wolfgang, 17

  Faust, 17

W

walnuts, 49, 106, 134, 201, 204–5, 228, 255
water consumption, 24, 81, 166
water exercise classes, 53
watermelon, 63, 117, 127, 196, 199, 252
water retention, 41–42, 194
Water Retention, 41
Weight Watchers, 34, 44
whey protein, 50, 72, 219
white coat hypertension, 108
wound healing, 33, 48, 75, 80, 82, 146, 152, 234, 241
Wound Healing, 151

Y

Yeast Connection, The (Crook), 183

Z

zeaxathin, 127
zinc, 61, 74, 241–42